KT-519-858

Women and the Health Care Industry

Buckingham: Open University   0335094724

GC 030214   GRIMSBY COLLEGE

WOMEN AND THE HEALTH CARE INDUSTRY
An Unhealthy Relationship?

GRIMSBY COLLEGE
LIBRARY
NUNS CORNER, GRIMSBY

Peggy Foster

OPEN UNIVERSITY PRESS
Buckingham · Philadelphia

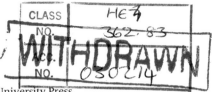
CLASS HE4
NO. 362·83
ACC. NO. 030214
WITHDRAWN

Open University Press
Celtic Court
22 Ballmoor
Buckingham
MK18 1XW

and
1900 Frost Road, Suite 101
Bristol, PA 19007, USA

First Published 1995

Copyright © Peggy Foster 1995

All rights reserved. Except for the quotation of short passages for the purpose of
criticism and review, no part of this publication may be reproduced, stored in a
retrieval system, or transmitted, in any form or by any means, electronic, mechanical,
photocopying, recording or otherwise, without the prior written permission of the
publisher or a licence from the Copyright Licensing Agency Limited. Details of such
licences (for reprographic reproduction) may be obtained from the Copyright
Licensing Agency Ltd of 90 Tottenham Court Road, London, W1P 9HE.

A catalogue record of this book is available from the British Library

ISBN   0 335 09472 4 (pb)   0 335 09473 2 (hb)

Library of Congress Cataloging-in-Publication Data
Foster, Peggy.
    Women and the health care industry : an unhealthy relationship? / Peggy Foster.
      p.   cm.
    Includes bibliographical references and index.
    ISBN 0-335-09472-4 (pbk.). — ISBN 0-335-09473-2
    1. Women's health services. 2. Medicine—Philosophy. 3. Women—Health and
hygiene—Sociological aspects. 4. Sexism in medicine. 5. Physician and patient. I.
Title.
RA564.85.F67   1995
362.1'98—dc20   94–42684
                                                                        CIP

Typeset by Type Study, Scarborough
Printed in Great Britain by Biddles Ltd, Guildford and King's Lynn

CONTENTS

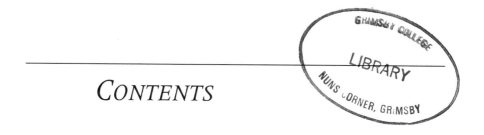

GRIMSBY COLLEGE
LIBRARY
NUNS CORNER, GRIMSBY

ACKNOWLEDGEMENTS

My colleagues in the School of Social Policy at the University of Manchester are more like a family to me than just people with whom I work. It seems invidious to pick out some colleagues for special thanks but Paul Wilding gave me a lot of fatherly support whilst I was writing this book and Duncan Scott reduced my teaching load just when I needed it most. Enid Roberts and Elaine Lewis have mothered me through good times and bad. Jen Dale, Karen Clarke, Trish Carabine and Jackie Boardman have all been like good sisters to me. But a special thanks must go to Jackie Boardman who shared the hard work of producing this book on a more or less daily basis, and whose skills and patience deserve a far greater reward than this acknowledgement. Thanks too to Alison Foulkes and Pauline Hollingsworth.

Most of the research for this book was done in libraries, so I would like to thank the most helpful and patient staff of the EOC information centre, Manchester, the John Rylands Library, the University of Manchester and the Women's Health and Reproductive Rights Information Centre, London.

Many authors acknowledge the support and patience of their partners and children but my special thanks for looking after me go to Paul Wilson for his practical and emotional support, Bob Cooke and June Brereton for enabling me to feel better than OK, my wonderful lodger Deirdre Doogan and my cousin Sarah Bartlett whose love and support never wavered even when I was being particularly difficult.

Finally, I would like to thank my publishers, Open University Press and Joan Malherbe in particular, for their patience whilst waiting – and waiting – for this book to be completed.

INTRODUCTION

The study of women and health care raises a whole range of challenging issues. A class of part time undergraduate students recently taught me a great deal about our responses to these issues. This highly intelligent and strongly motivated group were very open to the idea that modern medicine could sometimes be seen as a form of social or patriarchal control over women. They were also very prepared to consider critiques of modern medicine which focused on problems within the doctor–patient relationship. They were, however, far less ready to accept any evidence which indicated that modern medicine might be relatively ineffective or even harmful. We all want to believe that we can eat, drink and be merry for tomorrow the doctor will make sure we don't die. Acknowledging that doctors only rarely possess such magic powers can be extremely discomforting. Nevertheless the key theme of this book will be that women's consumption of health care is far less beneficial to them than is generally believed. This book will also claim that the current health care system in Great Britain benefits those who work in it or for it more than its consumers.

The idea that vested interests, including the very powerful interests of big business, play a key role in shaping the British health care system may seem strange to supporters of the National Health Service, very few of whom will readily associate it with the word industry which appears in the title of this book. Indeed, since its creation in 1948, the NHS has been resolutely defended by feminists amongst many others as a shining beacon of collectivist ideals and practices in a world increasingly dominated by rampant individualism and private markets. According to Rudolf Klein, the NHS was created as an act of faith and until very recently continued to be regarded by many of its supporters as a moral enterprise akin to a church. Klein cites Barbara Castle, speaking in the 1970s, who claimed 'intrinsically the National Health Service is a church. It is the nearest thing to the embodiment of the Good Samaritan that we have in any aspect of our public policy' (Castle in Klein 1993: 137).

If the National Health Service is a church then its most faithful congregation is predominantly a female one. The Office of Health Economics has calculated that in the mid-1980s women comprised 51 per cent of the UK population but consumed between 60 and 65 per cent of all NHS resources (Office of Health Economics 1987). Women visited their GPs almost twice as often as men; consumed more drugs and medicines than men; occupied acute hospital beds slightly more than men and were admitted to psychiatric units more than men (Kane 1991). Given such figures it is perhaps surprising that more men have not complained that the NHS allocates its resources unfairly in relation to gender. Probably most men assume, as do virtually all health care analysts, that women have an innate need for their larger share of health care resources. Indeed a whole range of theories has been developed to explain women's greater use of health care services. For some medical experts the answer clearly lies in women's biology. Women's complex reproductive systems, particularly their unique propensity to become pregnant and give birth are frequently cited as a self evident physiological explanation of women's apparent overuse of health care resources. According to Penny Kane, for example, 'the major reason that women use hospitals more than men is to do with their different biology. The female reproductive system is more complex and offers more possibilities for malfunction than the male one' (Kane 1991: 66). Another biologically deterministic explanation of women's excessive use of health care rests on the view that women's hormones and their fluctuating instability create women's unique vulnerability to a range of apparently emotional disturbances from PMS through postnatal depression to menopausal madness (see Ussher 1989).

A number of feminist writers have strongly criticized this biological model of women's vulnerability to ill health and particularly to mental health problems. In particular, feminists have emphasized the many ways in which a patriarchal society can literally make women sick. For example, feminists have suggested that postnatal depression is much less a hormonal imbalance than a perfectly natural, logical response to the overwhelming responsibility of motherhood in a society which provides mothers with so little financial, practical or even emotional support (Ussher 1989: Ch. 4).

At first sight the biological and feminist models of women's need for health care seem to be completely at odds with one another. However, in one sense both models share a common perspective. Both assume that it is women who rely relatively heavily on health care providers rather than vice versa. In both models the medical profession is seen as responding to a genuine need for health care. A key theme of this book will be that any dependency relationship between women and health care providers is at least partly the other way round. In other words all those employed in the manufacture and delivery of health care need women to consume their wares as much as, if not more than, women need the type of products and services they promote. If we begin to see the NHS in this way we may well have to stop using the metaphor of a church and instead regard the NHS more like a business or industry with a primary goal of attracting large numbers of customers and persuading them to use its services and products.

This claim may seem rather strange, if not heretical, to readers brought up to regard the National Health Service as an altruistic enterprise dedicated to meeting the needs of its patients. It may also seem odd to claim that the NHS is similar to a business trying to attract customers when traditionally it has been notorious for its long waiting lists and delays in providing treatment. Yet the idea that those providing health care need patients more than patients need them is certainly not an original one. In 1975 Ivan Illich claimed that the medical profession had become 'a major threat to health' (Illich 1975). In *Medical Nemesis* Illich argued that laymen were being disabled by their doctors both physically, emotionally and even socially. Illich backed up this claim by a wealth of evidence documenting the iatrogenic effects of modern medicine. Illich's argument that doctors were involved in an empire building exercise on the grandest of scales intrigued me when I first read it in the mid-1970s but at the time I quite failed to see that Illich's critique of the medical profession might be particularly relevant to doctors' relationships with women patients.

Within just a few years of the publication of *Medical Nemesis* however, the US women's health movement had begun to publish their own feminist critiques of male dominated modern medicine, some of which even outdid Illich in their total rejection of the benefits of late twentieth century health care systems. For example, in 1978 Mary Daly's *Gyn/Ecology* launched a blistering attack on a patriarchal medical profession. According to Daly, one of the most radical of radical feminists, American gynaecologists in the late twentieth century were mutilating and destroying women through their medical treatments. Daly argued that there was

> every reason to see the mutilation and destruction of women by doctors specializing in unnecessary radical mastectomies and hysterectomies, carcinogenic hormone therapy, psychosurgery, spirit-killing psychiatry and other forms of psychotherapy as directly related to the rise of radical feminism in the twentieth century.
>
> (1978: 228)

In other words Daly accused male doctors of waging an outright war against women in the name of patriarchy. For Daly male dominated modern medicine was of no benefit whatsoever to the women caught in its violent grip.

Very few feminists dismiss all modern medicine as iconoclastically as Mary Daly. Nevertheless, by the late 1970s a growing body of American feminist health care literature was beginning to challenge both the motives and methods of those 'high tech' medical priests who offered late twentieth century women medical salvation in response to all their day to day health and welfare problems. American feminists backed up their challenge with an impressive range of evidence documenting both the false promises held out by modern medicine and its damaging side effects. For example, in 1977 *Seizing Our Bodies*, edited by Claudia Dreifus and written by a collection of American feminists, contained essays on 'The dangers of contraception' by Barbara Seaman, 'The epidemic in unnecessary hysterectomy' by Deborah Larned and 'The theft of childbirth' by Adrienne Rich. Not only did this work question the patriarchal attitudes of male doctors towards their female patients, it also drew readers' attention to the very large sums of money to be made from the medicalization of American women's lives. For example, Deborah Larned suggested that at least some American gynaecologists advised women to have unnecessary hysterectomies because within the American fee-for-service health care system hysterectomies were an easy way for doctors to make money. Larned cited a Professor of Preventative Medicine who argued

> It seems inevitable that in any occupation where considerable income is available on the basis of events called operations a small percentage of people can well identify this as a marvelous income-producing device ... medicine is one of the few fields where if your wife wants a new coat, all you have to do is a couple more hysterectomies and she can buy it.
>
> (1977: 203)

Whilst American feminists have strongly attacked the exploitative nature of the American health care system British feminist health care analysts have focused far less on health care as a form of commercial exploitation of women. One reason for this is that those working within the NHS have indeed been far less dominated by a drive for financial gain than those working in the much more privatized US health care system. Another reason may be that British feminism has strong links with socialism and British socialists have always felt a sense of pride and ownership in the NHS. That is not to say that feminists writing about the British health care system have completely ignored the links between the NHS and capitalism. For example, in *The Political Economy of Health* Lesley Doyal (1979) suggested that one reason for the 'interventionist tendency' in modern obstetrics in Britain was that medical equipment manufacturers encouraged doctors to acquire the latest equipment. However, Doyal's main critique of the NHS in relation to women focused strongly on male doctors' patriarchal, sexist attitudes towards their female patients.

A focus on the doctor–patient relationship and the ideology of a male dominated medical profession is a particularly strong theme within British feminist analyses of health care. For example, in *The Patient Patients* Helen Roberts (1985) criticized the sexist/patriarchal ideology of women displayed both in the medical literature and in male doctors' actual practice. Similarly Ann Oakley, probably the most well known feminist health care writer in

Britain, has written brilliantly about the construction of a medical model of pregnancy and pregnant women and the way in which that model permeates obstetrical practice – tending to reduce women during pregnancy and labour to reproductive machines or at least to particularly passive patients (see Oakley 1980). Whilst Oakley has also been strongly critical of the spread of unnecessary obstetrical and antenatal 'high tech' interventions to perfectly normal healthy women her main theme has been the issue of who controls childbirth today rather than who profits from it in any commercial sense.

This book will also examine the relationship between doctors and their female patients and the key issue, which arises from that relationship, of who controls women's health care. However, its main focus will be on whether or not modern medicine is effective in relation to women's health needs and the extent to which ineffective and even dangerous medical interventions are promoted and perpetuated because of the many vested interests involved in their continued expansion.

In writing this book I have drawn heavily on US and British feminist critiques of a wide range of health care activities from contraception services (Chapter 1) through maternity care (Chapter 2) and new reproductive technologies (Chapter 3) to medical treatment of the menopause (Chapter 4) and the mental health care services for women (Chapter 5). In all these areas feminists have already mounted a strong challenge to the assumed effectiveness and safety of medical interventions. In other areas however British feminists have, on the whole, accepted the dominant medical view of particular interventions. For example, most British feminists accept that cancer screening programmes aimed at women are potentially life saving but agree with many doctors that they need to be better organized and resourced (Chapter 6). Feminists have been very critical of the manner in which cervical smear testing has been carried out and in particular they have strongly objected to the stigmatizing and punitive attitudes displayed by some doctors towards women whose smear tests have proved positive. Most feminists have not however seriously questioned the innate value of cancer screening tests. Similarly feminist health workers and writers have strongly objected to attempts by some medical experts to blame women for the spread of HIV infection and to stigmatize HIV positive women. But feminists have not yet seriously challenged the dominant medical view that HIV alone causes AIDS (Chapter 8). Indeed many feminist health care activists have been at the forefront of campaigns to inform women of this 'fact'. In other areas of health promotion feminists have again strongly objected to women-blaming approaches. They have, for example, combated the view that poor women choose unhealthy diets out of ignorance or laziness. They have not however challenged the dominant medical consensus on what constitutes a so-called healthy diet (Chapter 7). This book does challenge all these dominant medical assumptions. One of its central themes therefore, will be that much contemporary health care, including health promotion activities, is intrinsically more harmful to women than beneficial, whether or not it is delivered in a patronizing or sexist manner.

Most doctors offer their advice and treatments to women in the belief that what they have to offer is highly beneficial. Nevertheless, women need to bear in mind that even within the NHS health care providers will probably have a strong vested interest in their particular type of medical intervention. They are not therefore in the best position to evaluate those interventions with complete impartiality. A vested interest in a particular type of treatment need not just be pecuniary. Many doctors working full time in the NHS are undoubtedly dedicated to their work and do not seek particularly high levels of remuneration for the very high levels of commitment and sheer hard work they display. They would not be human however if they did not wish to gain some personal satisfaction from their work and therefore resisted evidence that their interventions were relatively ineffective or even harmful. It is hard to see how a doctor could gain any job satisfaction, if she or he genuinely believed that the service she or he was providing might be worse than useless. The same principle applies to other health care workers including the growing number of people working in the field of health promotion.

Sceptics of the efficacy of modern medical interventions have noted a tendency for supporters of those interventions to cite favourable research evidence indicating their effectiveness whilst conveniently ignoring other research studies which show no such benefits. Similarly the sceptics have claimed that medical journals show a strong tendency to publish articles which appear to demonstrate that a new drug or medical technique does work whilst rejecting more disappointing research findings. Indeed this tendency is so well ingrained within the world of medical research that many researchers simply fail to write up and submit negative results for publication (see Skrabanek and McCormick 1989). This type of medical bias has been clearly demonstrated in relation to AIDS research. Once the medical and scientific community had collectively decided that HIV was the sole cause of AIDS scientists whose research challenged that view found it extremely difficult to obtain funding to continue their research and almost impossible to get their views published in academic medical journals.

In this book any bias in the citing of research findings will be in favour of the sceptics. Whilst I have attempted to present a summary in each chapter of the dominant medical view of the topic being discussed, I have given most space to the views of the critics of modern medical interventions. The case for the effectiveness of, for example, antenatal screening or breast cancer screening is so widely available, both in health promotion literature and in popular women's magazines and newspapers, that I make no apology for giving more space to a critical perspective on modern medicine throughout this book. Ironically, whilst the general public is still being fed a predominantly optimistic view of the triumphs of modern medicine, a relatively superficial review of a range of serious medical journals quickly reveals a significant body of medical doubt and questioning in relation to a wide range of drugs, surgical procedures, screening programmes and even health promotion activities, which remains almost totally hidden from most laypersons' eyes. Thus, whilst much of the material presented in the following chapters owes a lot to previous feminist critiques of modern medicine, a fair proportion of the evidence against modern medical techniques has come directly from the research and writing of doctors themselves.

There are a number of noticeable gaps in the topics covered by this book. Given more time and space I would certainly have written more about gynaecological surgery, mental health care services – particularly the treatment of women suffering from psychotic illnesses – and modern medicine's response to the health problems of frail elderly women. These issues are certainly important but one has to stop somewhere! The other gap in my analysis was more deliberate. The book says relatively little about the key differences in women's experiences of health care which are determined by their class and ethnic origin. Variations in women's own experiences of health care will be examined in relation to the issue of modern medicine as a form of social control, and wherever sufficient evidence exists to back up a claim that certain groups of women have been targeted as recipients of medical care or advice as a form of social control, this evidence will be presented (see especially Chapter 1 and Chapter 3). However, the commonly heard feminist demand that far more health care resources should be specifically devoted to the needs of working-class and black women will not form a part of this book. Since one of its key themes will be that much contemporary health care actually does women more harm than good, it would clearly be illogical for it to demand that the most oppressed groups of women should be encouraged to use such health care more intensively. Finally, I have refrained from assuming that all women from ethnic minority groups can be grouped together as being more victimized by a white, male dominated health care system where no empirical evidence exists to demonstrate this. I have therefore refrained from adding 'and of course it is much worse for black women' at the end of any particular piece of critical analysis.

I want to stress at this point that this book is not intended to dictate to women exactly what they should or should not do to meet their own health needs. Books which insist that women should eschew all things conventionally medical on the grounds that modern medicine is lethal are in many ways as misleading as the worst form of medical evangelism. Books on alternative health care which promise perfect health and well-being to women who adopt rigid diets or punitive exercise routines are frequently both impractical and deceptive. In any case, most women will always seek expert medical advice and help of some kind, in the hope of finding a solution to debilitating or even life threatening health problems. Even if a mass withdrawal from the consumption of modern medicine might, on balance, do women more good than harm, it is a completely unrealistic goal. The main message of this book is not therefore that women must avoid all forms of modern medicine, but rather that women need to become much more sceptical and better informed health care consumers. They need to be as wary of claims made for a new medical product or surgical treatment as they are over claims that a new soap powder will wash whiter than white. In fact, given the potentially dangerous side effects of most modern medical interventions, women need to be even more wary when considering a medical treatment than when selecting products off a supermarket shelf.

More information about the relative ineffectiveness and possible harmful side effects of a whole range of modern medical interventions may upset those women who are used to placing great faith in their doctors. However, such information can be empowering. The more information which women receive on the costs to them of relying so heavily on the health care industry, the more likely they may be to become active rather than passive consumers of this industry's wares. It is this goal of empowering women health care consumers which lies behind the writing of this book.

1

CONTRACEPTION AND ABORTION

Contraceptive pills, IUDs, diaphragms and caps, long term injectables, implants, sheaths of all colours and flavours, a sponge full of spermicide, sterilization, books on natural methods of contraception and, if all that fails, a morning-after pill or a safe, legal abortion – the late twentieth century is undoubtedly perceived as an era of choice and opportunity for women who wish to regulate their fertility.

Presumably, therefore, women today should be extremely grateful to the inventors and purveyors of modern forms of fertility control on the grounds that they have liberated women from a form of biological tyranny? This is certainly the view taken by some male experts on women and reproduction. It is not, however, a view universally held by women themselves. Some women have overtly questioned the motives of modern family planners and have become increasingly sceptical of their apparently safe and efficacious wares. In this chapter we will outline the medical model of contraception before critically evaluating that model, not only in terms of the safety and effectiveness of modern forms of contraception, but also in terms of who exercises control over their usage.

The development of contraceptive services

Until the mid to late twentieth century, most women's lives were dominated by their reproductive systems. Lacking access to effective, safe forms of contraception and unable to refuse husbands their conjugal rights, most fertile women throughout the ages could not avoid the dangerous and debilitating treadmill of all too frequent pregnancies and childbirths. If any woman today imagines that a woman's reproductive life was more natural and less controlled in previous times, she would do well to read Edward Shorter's *A History of Women's Bodies* (1984) wherein the fear, pain, disease and death so commonly associated with traditional childbirths are portrayed in almost unbearably graphic detail. Some feminist historians have argued that before the rise of the modern, predominantly male, medical profession, wise women were the experts on pregnancy, childbirth and contraception and that women themselves controlled what knowledge there was about natural herbal remedies for female maladies, knowledge which was later suppressed and lost (see, for example, Ehrenreich and English 1979). Whilst accepting the feminist view of the rise of the modern medical profession as at least in part a patriarchal power struggle against women healers, I'm afraid the evidence which survives of the efficacy or acceptability of traditional 'wise woman' methods of fertility control is not impressive. Edward Shorter is clearly no feminist, but we have no reason to doubt his horrific accounts of natural childbirths which went wrong, or do-it-yourself abortions which not only failed to work but seriously endangered the woman's life. Shorter argues that by the early twentieth century women had gained significant reproductive freedoms, but other historical accounts clearly show that even by the late 1930s many working-class women's lives were still totally circumscribed by endless pregnancies and dire poverty (Spring-Rice 1981). In 1939, the results of a questionnaire on women's health sent to 1,250 working-class wives clearly demonstrated the very negative effects of too many pregnancies and births on these women's health and welfare (Spring-Rice 1981). Mrs W of East London, for example, had had 22 pregnancies by the age of 43 – 13 children and nine miscarriages. She had suffered from anaemia, kidney trouble and heart trouble for years and thought she had had 'rather too many children'. Mrs Y of South Wales had had five children in five years. Her health visitor commented

> Mrs Y looks in very poor condition, she says she always feels tired and disinclined to do anything. I think she was probably anaemic before marriage and five pregnancies in five years have drained her vitality.
>
> (Spring-Rice 1981: 53)

The author of the report commented that

> contraceptive advice seems practically non-existent. A few women . . . speak of having been to the Birth Control Clinics but there are dozens of women in obvious need of such advice either for procuring proper intervals between births or to have no more children, who, although they have been told by their doctor that this is necessary, are not instructed by him in scientific methods and do not go to a Birth Control Clinic even if

there is one within reach. This seems to indicate a deplorable ignorance or prejudice on the part of the professional medical attendant.

(Spring-Rice 1981: 44)

Such prejudice on the part of the medical profession played an important role in restricting women's access to information on birth control well into the late twentieth century. Histories of the development of birth control clinics in Britain show clearly how provision of contraceptive services slowly developed outside mainstream medicine. Family planning, for example, was not even mentioned during the long discussions between the government and the medical profession leading up to the creation of the NHS. During the 1950s the voluntary Family Planning Association (FPA) gradually expanded its clinics providing women with diaphragms and caps, but most married couples still relied – if they used anything at all – on condoms or withdrawal (Shapiro 1987: Ch. 2). Meanwhile, any sexually active single woman still faced the awful dilemma, if she became accidentally pregnant, of giving the baby away or facing an illegal, dangerous backstreet abortion unless, of course, she was rich enough to procure the services of a highly skilled private gynaecologist or lucky enough to escape into a 'shotgun' marriage.

It was the invention of 'the pill' which eventually revolutionized the medical profession's attitude towards providing their patients with contraceptive advice. In 1960, the first high dose combined steroid pill came on to the American market, having been first tested on a very small number of poor Puerto Rican women (Seaman 1978). Unlike previous methods of contraception, the pill could only be prescribed by a doctor and so the British medical profession, very reluctantly at first, began to play a much greater role in the provision of contraceptive services. By 1964, nearly half a million British women were taking high dose hormonal pills (Mosse and Heaton 1990: 59). By the end of the 'swinging 60s', the NHS (Family Planning) Act 1967 had made it possible for health authorities to provide contraception on NHS prescription, the FPA had deleted the mention of married women from its aims and the 1967 Abortion Act had given women very limited access to safe, legal abortions. At the time, women undoubtedly felt that they had a lot to gain from these developments. Germaine Greer, writing in 1984, recalls how she and her friends in the late 1960s vociferously demanded the pill from a reluctant medical profession (Greer 1984: 158). In the early 1970s, my contemporaries at a British university were also determined to gain access to this new wonder drug. I recall long debates about how best to persuade reluctant GPs to prescribe the pill to young, unmarried women, and angry tirades at 'fuddy-duddy' doctors who flatly refused to do so. Ironically, I do not recall any interest being expressed as to what was actually in the pill or how precisely it worked, it was just seized upon as part of a more general, revolutionary life plan which would liberate us from the narrow conventions and constrictions of our mothers' generation. It was also seized upon by young men who urged their girlfriends to 'go on the pill'.

Young women demanded the pill; doctors, often reluctantly at first, began to prescribe it for them. It is important to note, however, that a number of different interest groups were already clearly established. Many young people saw the pill as part of a sexual revolution. Family planners and many doctors were primarily concerned to find methods of contraception which could control a world wide population explosion and prevent 'unsuitable' women from having babies (see, for example, Yanoshik and Norsigian 1989). Pharmaceutical companies had their own agenda which was, as always, to produce products which would sell widely enough to generate large profits.

Although British women began being prescribed the pill in the mid-1960s, it was not until the mid-1970s that the current system of contraceptive services in Britain was finally in place. From 1975, GPs began to be paid a specific fee for providing a contraceptive service to individual patients. Since, at that time, most GPs had no training whatsoever in this field most of them only prescribed the pill which could be done, ironically, with no specific medical training. Fitting an IUD was too skilled a task for most GPs at that time, whilst handing out free condoms was apparently beneath the GPs' dignity and thus left to family planning clinics. These clinics were finally incorporated into the NHS in the mid-1970s and generally offered a much wider range of advice and services than those offered by GPs.

Contraception: the medical model

Although doctors clearly differ significantly amongst themselves in their attitudes towards contraception and women who require contraceptive services, a careful study of medical texts on contraception and abortion does reveal a dominant medical model which emphasizes the need for doctors to give women expert advice on fertility control and favours certain methods of contraception over others. Moreover, research studies have confirmed that many practising doctors are putting this textbook model into practice.

Recent research has found, for example, that GPs strongly prefer the pill when providing their patients with contraceptive services. A research report published in 1988 based on a study of over 60 clinics and GP surgeries in the south of England, found that the pill was prescribed by GPs 84 per cent of the time and 55 per cent of the time by doctors working in family planning clinics. GPs inserted IUDs in 10 per cent of cases compared to 23 per cent of clinic cases. Caps and diaphragms were provided only 2 per cent of the time by GPs and only 9 per cent of the time by clinics (Mosse and Heaton 1990: 70).

Why is the contraceptive pill so popular with doctors? There are a number of influences on doctors' contraceptive habits. First, the pill is relatively easy to prescribe. GPs need no special training to prescribe it and only quick and easy routine tests are deemed necessary before a woman is prescribed the pill for the first time. Second, contraceptive pills are also frequently advertised in journals distributed free to GPs, such as *Doctor*. Whilst full page glossy advertisements for particular brands of contraceptive pill are seen frequently in these magazines, advertisements for diaphragms are noticeable by their absence. Third, in order to insert IUDs and fit diaphragms, GPs need special training, but many GPs have not undertaken any such training (Mosse and Heaton 1990). Finally, medical textbooks, including textbooks aimed specifically at trainee GPs, tend strongly to support pill prescribing, particularly for certain groups of women. For example, in Loudon's *Handbook of Family Planning*, Reid advises doctors in a section on young people that 'a low dose oestrogen/progesterone pill is probably best for a girl whose periods are well established, provided she can be relied upon to take it regularly' (1985: 32). Despite recurrent scare stories in the press about the risks of long term pill usage, the medical profession appears to have few doubts about the pill's safety. Modern medical textbooks acknowledge that some women, including young women, are now increasingly concerned about the risks of long term pill taking, particularly the possible increased risk of cervical and breast cancer. The medical consensus appears to be, however, that women are unnecessarily worried about the potential risks. Guillebaud and Law, for example, have criticized the press for unnecessarily scaring women taking the pill: 'Exaggerated press reports can cause unjustified alarm, upsetting the equanimity of some patients who are happily using a certain method and preventing others from starting it' (1987: 123). Guillebaud and Law went on to argue that if the pill was in any way associated with an increased risk of cervical cancer it was merely 'at worst' a 'weak co-factor, possibly speeding transition through the pre-invasive stages', since 'the prime carcinogen is quite clearly sexually transmitted' (1987: 129).

Other medical experts on the pill have taken a similarly reassuring stance in relation to recurrent scares over the link with female cancers. For example, in 1989 when the press reported research linking long term pill use to an increased risk of breast cancer in younger women, Dr Clifford Kay, a leading medical authority on the pill, argued in *The Daily Express* (6 May 1989) that as far as he was concerned women in the study were 'probably close to developing breast cancer anyway. The pill had merely accelerated its arrival.' In *The Times* (5 June 1989) he emphasized that it was smoking that caused the real problems rather than pill usage *per se*: 'If you can exclude breast cancer and stop women smoking the pill is fantastically safe. All the major risks of heart attack and strokes are confined to women who smoke.'

Guillebaud and Law (1987) advise GPs that it can prove very reassuring to 'over-anxious' patients to show them a table of comparative risks which demonstrates amongst other comparisons that pill use is much, much safer than hang-gliding, coal mining, having a baby in Ecuador or even playing soccer – activities not routinely undertaken by the majority of fertile British women.

As well as dismissing women's fears about possible links between long term pill usage and cancer, some medical experts have also been dismissive of women's complaints of more minor side effects from contraceptive pill taking. For many years individual women who experienced very uncomfortable side effects when using high dosage pills were told they must be imagining things. Germaine Greer, for example, has recounted how, when she finally told her doctor in the late 1960s that she thought the pill must be causing her to burst into tears several times a day for no apparent reason, he simply told her that it couldn't be (Greer 1984). By the late 1980s some medical texts did list a very wide range of possible side effects which can be experienced by pill users. The *Handbook of Family Planning* (Loudon 1985), for example, does discuss the possibility of loss of libido, headaches, weight gain and other side effects related to the contraceptive pill. In most instances however, these problems are not deemed to be caused by the pill *per se*. For example, according to Guillebaud any weight gain which occurs on low dose pills is 'commonly due to overeating' (Guillebaud 1985: 68) whilst the finding that depression is commoner among women on the pill than non-pill users is, Guillebaud claims, probably due to 'the general life circumstances of the pill-taker rather than the pill itself' (1985: 66). Tindall's edition of *Jeffcoate's Principles of Gynaecology* is even more dismissive of the so-called minor side effects of the pill:

> Almost all the symptoms and ill effects that one can imagine have been and are credited to the pill and are used as an excuse for women, influenced by inspired and calculated adverse propaganda, to discontinue taking it. Controlled observations show that many of the alleged reactions are not in any way attributable to the hormones; they are either present before treatment is started or would have occurred anyway. Real and fictitious side effects described include the following . . .
>
> (Tindall 1987: 613)

There is also evidence that GPs providing contraceptive services ignore or reinterpret women's complaints about the negative side effects they experience whilst taking the contraceptive pill. One study of 50 middle-class British women carried out in the early 1980s found several instances where women who had complained to their doctor about the side effects they experienced whilst taking the pill found that he or she took no notice of them or reinterpreted the problem. One woman reported 'It was as if I was imagining them . . . It's almost as if they can't hear you'. Another, who was suffering from vaginal discharge complained 'I've tried to talk to them but you never seem to get anything but put-off replies like "Females always have a certain amount of infection in their vaginas"' (Pollock 1984: 146). The researcher concluded that doctors' opinions about the side effects and risks involved in using contraceptives were so definite that what women themselves said about their experiences 'made very little difference' (Pollock 1984: 145).

Whilst many doctors appear to dismiss or deflect women's own negative experiences of contraceptive use, the medical profession as a whole still appears to be reluctant to give women full information on both the potential long term risks and the known immediate side effects of hormonal forms of contraception.

When Jean Robinson, a lay member of the General Medical Council, was researching the possible causes of cervical cancer and found research data linking it to pill usage she was told by gynaecologists that they had not given women this information for fear that women might stop taking the pill (Hynes and Spallone 1990).

As well as defending the contraceptive pill from critics who regard it as a dangerous form of contraception overloaded with unpleasant side effects, members of the medical profession have also claimed that both injectable forms of hormonal contraception, such as Depo Provera and modern types of IUD are both safe and relatively painless to use. Whilst some doctors are not convinced about either of these forms of contraception, many medical texts and journal articles continue to recommend them and extol their safety. According to an editorial in *The Lancet* (28 March 1992) on IUDs the latest large scale research has found that there is only 'a slight risk of Pelvic Inflammatory Disease (PID) during the first days post-insertion and thereafter there is little difference between rates of IUD users and the background population' (p. 783). The editorial concluded that, for women 'in low risk groups, there seems to be little if any risk of getting PID with modern copper-releasing IUDs' (p. 784).

Medical confidence in the safety of injectable forms of hormonal contraceptives is also to be found in many medical texts. In the *Handbook of Family Planning*, for example, Elizabeth Wilson claims that

> It is probable that DMPA (Depo Provera) carries a lower risk of death and a lower morbidity rate than many other forms of contraception, such as the combined pill and the IUD. It should therefore be available to all women on the same basis as these other methods.
>
> (Wilson 1985: 117)

Guillebaud and Law in *Women's Problems in General Practice* argue that Depo Provera

> has been repeatedly endorsed by expert committees of prestigious bodies including WHO. Anxiety has been generated by animal research of very doubtful relevance to humans. A consensus view is that Depo Provera is actually a safer drug than the combined pill, despite the adverse publicity it receives.
>
> (Guillebaud and Law 1987: 146)

Some members of the medical profession also appear to believe that the amount of information about the side effects and risks of injectable contraceptives should vary according to the type of patient being counselled. According to the *Handbook of Family Planning*, for example, how much a doctor should tell a patient about the possible risks attached to injectable contraceptives 'must depend on his own judgement of the patient's intelligence and background' (Wilson 1985: 123).

Why is the medical profession as a whole so keen to defend the safety record of hormonal contraception, including controversial injectables? It seems clear that doctors are particularly keen on methods of contraception which leave them in control. They dislike methods which appear to them to be far too prone to user error and thus failure in terms of unwanted or accidental pregnancies. The majority of doctors do not apparently approve of early abortion as an alternative method of controlling the number of unwanted pregnancies. According to Rose Shapiro,

> The need of family planning organizations and doctors to prevent pregnancy is so powerful that it manifests itself almost as an irrational fear. The impression given is that accidental pregnancy is the worst thing that could ever happen to woman and that abortion is an absolute disaster.
>
> (Shapiro 1987: 41)

Doctors' concern to prevent unwanted or accidental pregnancies appears to be particularly important in relation to certain types of female patients. The *Handbook of Family Planning*, for example, counsels doctors that 'mini-pills are not generally recommended for teenagers for whom effective contraception is usually of prime importance' (Loudon 1985: 109). The *Handbook* therefore recommends the combined pill for young girls unless contraindicated or unless the girl cannot be relied upon to take it regularly. The diaphragm is ruled out for most of this age group on the grounds that 'they are often poorly motivated to use it reliably' (Reid 1985: 33). A gynaecologist writing in *The Practitioner* was in favour of 'selling' the combined pill to young women. 'The time has now come' he argued, 'to persuade young women to take the pill by emphasizing its 'non-contraceptive advantages' (Bowen-Simpkins 1988: 16).

While most medical experts regard the pill as a safe and highly effective form of contraception for 'well-motivated' women, including young women, some experts have argued that a small group of women may not be responsible enough to be relied upon to take the pill. Tindall's textbook on gynaecology, for example, advises that whilst IUDs are not to be preferred to oral contraceptives for the woman who is 'conscientious and intelligent', they are especially valuable in the cases of 'feckless and irresponsible women (and husbands) and for mental defectives and mental misfits' (Tindall 1987: 608). Similarly, Reid advises in the *Handbook of Family Planning* that for poorly motivated women

> who include the mothers of large families, of children in care or with very little care, those with haphazard personal and social relationships, in trouble with the law, and with substandard living conditions ...

Methods such as the IUD or the injectable which do not require the patient's co-operation are often best.

(Reid 1985: 36)

Bowen-Simpkins advised in *The Practitioner* (1988: 16): 'Occasionally an injectable may be recommended for a highly promiscuous teenager who is unreliable with other methods'.

Whilst most GPs seem happiest prescribing the pill for the great majority of their patients and even family planning clinics which specialize in offering a range of contraceptives will prescribe the pill to the majority of women attending them, most medical textbooks which discuss contraceptive methods do not appear to be overtly against barrier methods of contraception. In *Women's Problems in General Practice*, for example, the diaphragm is described as 'capable of excellent protection provided it is correctly and consistently used' (Guillebaud and Law 1987: 155). Yet, in practice, diaphragms are very rarely given to patients seeking contraception from either GPs or family planning clinics. There are probably several factors behind the relative unpopularity of diaphragms with the medical profession. First, they are not vigorously marketed to GPs in the same way as contraceptive pills. One GP has commented that in 1983, after the media publicized research linking the pill to both breast and cervical cancer, there was suddenly a 'rash of advertisements' in the medical press for 'caps, coils, jellies, creams'. She noted

General practitioners have always suffered from a lack of information about barrier methods of contraception and indeed are generally unwilling, possibly because of ignorance, to advise about and prescribe these methods. Many doctors regard the form for claiming for 'contraceptive services' as a 'pill' form. Here, however, we were suddenly bombarded with advertising material about non-hormonal methods.

(Yudkin 1984: 13)

Second, medical textbooks tend to stress that 'high motivation is essential if female barrier methods are to be successful'. They tend to advise doctors that such methods are best suited to women in 'stable partnerships' and that they are not suitable for younger unmarried women. Finally, doctors seem to believe that barrier methods, such as diaphragms and caps are not popular with women themselves. According to one consultant gynaecologist, for example,

the diaphragm is not popular with teenagers. This may in part be due to ignorance of the method but for many it is the fitting by a doctor or nurse that is too offputting. The premeditation involved is not appealing and the method may be considered messy. In my experience the girl seeking advice about the diaphragm is usually intelligent and accompanied by her partner.

(Bowen-Simpkins 1988: 16)

In summary, the dominant consensus within the medical profession appears to be that the pill, the coil and injectables are all safe and highly effective methods of contraception. They are also forms of contraception that do not require any high levels of skill or motivation on the part of the patient. This is very important because, for many doctors, women themselves cannot necessarily be relied upon to prevent unwanted pregnancies. They therefore need the skilled advice and help of doctors who will be able to judge which particular type of contraceptive is best suited to which type of woman. Most medical experts admit that no method of contraception is perfect and that most of the methods they prefer do have some negative side effects. Again, however, the medical consensus appears to be that many women tend to exaggerate the side effects of contraception and subjectively attribute problems such as weight gain or depression to their contraceptive method rather than their own lifestyles or emotional makeup.

The above view of contraception is quite overt and easily found in widely used medical texts and journals. The link between medical contraceptive services and profit taking is, however, much more hidden. Textbooks for trainee GPs certainly do not advise them which contraceptive methods will make most money for their practices. Advertisements for new contraceptive pills in medical journals do not, of course, indicate how much profit the manufacturers hope to make from their new product. Very occasionally, however, glimpses of the links between money making and contraceptive services can be found. In a free magazine distributed to GPs entitled *Financial Pulse* (22 May 1990), for example, GPs were advised that 'the key to profiting from contraception lies in realizing that there is more to it than simple drug prescription'. GPs were then reminded that, whilst the government would only pay them £12.30 a year for prescribing the pill, they could earn up to £42.25 for fitting an IUD. So far this disparity in financial incentives has not led to doctors abandoning their strong preference for the pill but it does clearly indicate that the provision of contraceptive services can be a profitable exercise even for doctors working wholly within the NHS whose patients pay nothing directly for the services they receive. It is equally important to recognize that drugs companies make large profits by supplying contraceptive pills to the NHS. Prescriptions for the pill currently cost the NHS over £3 million per annum. When in 1993 the government announced its intention to limit the range of contraceptive pills provided on the NHS to the less expensive brands, drugs companies understandably fought back and suggested that if this measure was implemented they might 'pull out of the market' and discontinue their research into new safer and more effective pills (*Doctor*, 1 April 1993). Doctors also complained that if women had to obtain the more expensive pills privately, they might have to pay up to £20 a month. This figure gives some indication of the hidden profits behind women's consumption of contraceptive pills. The manufacture and sale of IUDs is also highly profitable. In the early 1970s the American company Robins made huge profits by heavily promoting the Dalkon Shield IUD before it was withdrawn from the market having caused at least 20 deaths in the United States alone and tens of thousands of injuries to women worldwide (Yanoshik and Norsigian 1989). Significantly, high sales of the Dalkon Shield occurred after Dr Hugh J. Davis had published his book *The Intrauterine Device for Contraception* (Davis 1971 cited by Dowie and Johnston 1978) which advised doctors that the IUD was much safer than the pill. On every graph and chart in this book the Dalkon Shield came out top in terms of safety and efficiency. What the book did not say, however, was that its author had invented the Dalkon Shield. Before the Shield was finally removed from the market, Davis would earn more than half a million dollars in relation to it (Dowie and Johnston 1978). This particular scandal has understandably led to some scepticism from women who are now reassured by the medical profession that today's IUDs are extremely safe and reliable. Undoubtedly, most doctors prescribing contraceptives within the NHS are not consciously profit-driven and are genuinely concerned to meet the needs of their female patients as effectively and as safely as possible. Their preference for hormonal forms of contraception, for example, certainly cannot be explained solely in terms of profit-hungry pill manufacturers using the medical profession as 'pill pushers'. Nevertheless, it is important to bear in mind the link between contraception and profit making when assessing the claims of supporters of the more medicalized and expensive forms of contraceptive wares.

Modern contraception: a critical evaluation

The safety of contraceptives

Whilst their manufacturers and the majority of the medical profession continue to insist that modern forms of contraception are extremely safe and effective and relatively free from unpleasant side effects, some feminists have claimed that the pill and other medicalized forms of contraception are so dangerous that women should totally avoid them. For example, an article in *Spare Rib* in 1990 stated boldly

> of course oral contraceptives are dangerous and pose a risk to women who take them. No amount of scrupulous testing is going to make them better ... 30 years after the introduction of the Pill, the reality is that whatever ease it comes packaged with the hazards and risks are too high.
>
> (Hynes and Spallone 1990: 49)

The article cited research linking contraceptive pill taking with an increased risk of breast cancer and it is this possible link which worries many women who are now, or who ever have been, pill users. Unfortunately, it is extremely difficult to make any definitive statements about links between the pill and the risks of cancer. It does appear that taking the pill actually protects women to some extent from cancer of the endometrium (lining of the womb) and cancer of the ovaries (which is as common as cervical cancer; see Hayman 1993). On the other hand, several research studies published during the 1980s demonstrated a link between pill use and breast and cervical cancer in younger women. For example, research published in 1983 found an increased risk of breast cancer for young women who had taken the pill before they were 25 (Pike *et al.*, 1983). Since then, despite attempts by some medical experts to discredit these research findings, other research studies have also found an increased risk of breast cancer among younger women who took the pill for several years before their first pregnancy. A study published in 1989 found that, whilst the risk of developing breast cancer among non-pill taking women under the age of 36 was about one in 500, that risk rose to one in 300 amongst women who had taken the pill for four to eight years (Chilvers *et al.*, 1989). Despite the worrying significance of these findings, the Medical Research Council actually withdrew funding from this research project, and research proposed by the Royal College of General Practitioners into pill use in 120,000 women was also denied funding by the MRC (*New Woman*, April 1992). Meanwhile, *crucially* we still do not know whether there may be a link between pill taking in early adulthood and the development of breast cancer much later in life. Given this frightening gap in our knowledge – the pill has been called 'the largest uncontrolled experiment in human carcinogenesis ever known' (Epstein cited by Phillips and Rakusen 1989: 541) – and given growing evidence of a link between pill use and breast cancer in younger women, it is surely at the very least worrying that young women are still not receiving full information about this risk. For example, *The Family Planning Association Guide to Contraception* (1993) claims that the pill protects women against cancer of the endometrium and ovaries but makes absolutely no mention of any increased risk of breast or cervical cancer (Hayman 1993). It is also disturbing to see similar reassurances being given about Depo Provera and other injectable forms of contraception. In 1993 *The Family Planning Association Guide to Contraception*, for example, stated 'There are no serious illnesses linked to using injectable contraception' and claimed that any side effects that a user might experience 'are likely to be mild and short-lived' (Hayman 1993: 43).

In 1992 a large scale WHO study did report that there was no evidence to suggest any increased risk of cervical cancer in women using Depo Provera long term (Thomas and Ray 1992) but previous smaller studies had reported just such a risk. In 1990 an American study reported a 2.4 times increased risk of cervical cancer in women using injectables for five years or more compared with controls (Herrero 1990). In 1989 a study published in the *British Medical Journal* found that women who had breast cancer diagnosed between the ages of 25 and 34 were twice as likely as the controls to have used Depo Provera (Paul *et al.* 1989).

Whilst the risk of dying from using medicalized forms of modern contraception such as the pill and Depo Provera are undoubtedly extremely small, some women have found that, despite reassurances from their doctors, the side effects from these contraceptive methods have been so unpleasant that they have given up using them. One woman, for example, has recounted 'I felt fat and lethargic using the Pill. The doctor said that it had nothing to do with it. I changed to a diaphragm on a friend's advice and lost a lot of weight and felt healthier' (Oxford Women's Health Action Group 1984: 31). Ironically, some women have noted a loss of libido whilst taking the pill. One woman who asked her doctor if there was any chance the pill was affecting her libido was told 'it was more likely time to change partners' (Mosse and Heaton 1990: 277). It must be emphasized that some women have nothing but praise for the pill – for example: 'I have only used the pill. It was simple for me to use and I had no side effects whatsoever' and 'I've had no trouble at all and I chose it because of its reliability and the lack of fuss involved' (Oxford Women's Health Action Group 1984: 30). Such consumer satisfaction, however, is no reason for doctors failing to give all women adequate information about possible side effects and for not taking seriously those women who do experience problems. The issue of side effects is particularly important in relation to injectable hormonal contraceptives and implants, since it is harder to stop their effects immediately than it is to stop taking a daily swallowed pill. Opponents of Depo Provera have claimed that far from being 'mild', the side effects of this type of contraception can sometimes be very severe. According to Phillida Bunkle, for example, although the medical literature does usually acknowledge that 'bleeding disturbances' are a common side effect of Depo Provera it does not acknowledge how disabling these disturbances can be and the dangers of heavy bleeding have been 'consistently minimised' by its manufacturers Upjohn. Bunkle argues that research studies funded by Upjohn have ignored women's own accounts of the severity of the side effects of Depo Provera. She quotes one user as reporting 'Within 24 hours of the injection I started bleeding. I flooded for 14 weeks. In that time I lost 3 stone . . . I couldn't go out. Sometimes I could only crawl around' (Bunkle 1984: 177). In 1992, the *Women's Health Newsletter* reported the concerns of a women's health group in a large inner city area in the north of England who had encountered a number of women on Depo Provera who were suffering from heavy bleeding and weight gain after having been given no warning that such side effects are quite common (Bastias 1992: 12). Yet, when a government appeal panel decided to grant the manufacturers of Depo Provera a long term British licence, they referred to the drug having 'common and unpleasant side effects' (Lister 1984: 13) and recommended that heavy bleeding should be clearly stated as an adverse effect on the drug's data sheet. The panel also concluded that Depo Provera had not been subject to good quality epidemiological research and criticized its manufacturers Upjohn for not giving sufficient weight to 'short term risks' but they nevertheless granted them the licence Upjohn sought (Lister 1984). No doubt the panel assumed that in future women would be able to make an informed choice over whether or not to take Depo Provera but this is just what many women cannot do, since powerful vested interests cannot or will not accept that all women should be treated as intelligent, responsible adults who are entitled to decide for themselves whether the potential side effects of the more medicalized forms of modern contraception outweigh their undoubted benefit in terms of effectively preventing unplanned pregnancies.

Contraception as social control

Feminists have not only expressed their concern over the physical side effects of modern forms of contraception, they have also strongly objected to those doctors and family planners who see a role for contraception as a form of social control over certain types of women. Black feminists in particular have accused the medical profession of combining racism and sexism in stereotyping black women as undesirable mothers and unreliable contraceptive users. For example, according to Bryan *et al.*:

> Black women's ability to reproduce has come to be viewed as a moral flaw, to be frowned upon and controlled – so much so that doctors frequently take it upon themselves to exercise control over our fertility in the interests of (white) society. The consequences of this are evident in the numerous cases of Black women who receive unwanted sterilizations or terminations, or the damaging long-term contraceptive DP (Depo Provera) all in the interests of controlling the numbers of 'unwanted' Black babies ... Many paternal and apparently sympathetic doctors have persuaded Black women to accept an abortion or contraceptive she did not really want, out of a concern to control our fertility ... There are a lot of doctors who don't even bother to make a secret of the fact that they go along with the idea that we are sapping their country's resources and see it as their professional duty to keep our numbers down. They say things like 'Well you've already got two children, so why do you need to have any more? You might as well get your tubes tied when you come in for that D&C'. It's only when you hear Black women talking and realize how many of us this is happening to that you see things in perspective.
>
> (1985: 103)

Many black women and white working-class women, particularly single mothers, are very vulnerable to poverty and deprivation and this often has a negative impact on their children. Yet, rather than tackling these problems directly, society appears to prefer the much cheaper option of more effective family planning services targeted at the poor and deprived. Women living in poverty are thus sometimes labelled by health and welfare professionals as 'poor mothers' and 'encouraged' to use the 'most effective' forms of contraception.

To the medical profession, sometimes genuinely frustrated by some women's 'reckless' incapacity to use effectively contraceptives such as the diaphragm or the pill, injectable and implantable contraceptives may offer a wonderful opportunity to dispense with the need for daily patient cooperation and compliance in preventing unwanted pregnancies. To some feminists, on the other hand, injectable and implantable contraceptives are the most extreme form of medical control over women's fertility. Women they fear, particularly deprived women, are being used by family planners as guinea pigs in a mass experiment to solve the world's population problem. According to Janet Hadley, a strong opponent of Depo Provera, for example, 'Population control is the opposite of what the women's liberation movement stands for. Population control relies on drugs and devices whose side effects and risks are concealed from their users' (1987: 173).

The latest form of contraception which some feminists fear may be used in an overtly controlling way in Britain is Norplant which was licensed for use in the UK in the summer of 1993. Whilst a number of doctors and family planners have welcomed this new type of hormonal contraceptive as an expansion of women's choice, critics have pointed out that Norplant has already been used in extremely coercive ways in the United States. In January 1991, an American judge gave a woman convicted of beating her children the choice of a longer prison sentence or release on probation on condition that she accepted Norplant (Platt 1991). In 1992 a state senator, Walter Graham, proposed a bill that would have made Norplant mandatory for any woman in Mississippi with four or more children who wanted any kind of government welfare (*New Woman*, September 1993). According to Julie Mertus, these uses of Norplant 'far from being part of a new trend hark ... back to old-fashioned eugenics: plans to "improve" society by ensuring that "undesirables" do not reproduce' (Mertus, cited by Platt 1991).

Since Norplant is only just becoming available for use in Britain, we clearly do not have any evidence of it being used in a coercive or overtly controlling way in relation to British women. However, given the tide of moral panic generated in the early 1990s against single young mothers living on benefit and calls for welfare benefits to be restricted to women with just one child, it may well not be long before some right-wing politician suggests that single mothers on income support should agree to Norplant as a condition of receiving further benefits. Yet magazines aimed at young women have welcomed Norplant as 'the perfect contraception' for them (*The Clothes Show Magazine*, September 1993). A more accurate description of Norplant can be found in *Doctor*, a free journal distributed within the medical profession only, which listed Norplant's side effects as irregular bleeding, headaches, nervousness, acne and weight gain but also noted its key advantage – 'compliance is guaranteed' (*Doctor*, 14 January 1993).

Abortion

As we noted earlier one motive behind doctors' emphasis on the efficacy as opposed to the safety of the contraceptives they prescribe is their strong motivation to reduce women's demands for abortions. Yet women themselves may well have a very different perspective on the priority which should be given to preventing unplanned pregnancies when choosing a method of contraception. For example, when Margaret Pyke and Marie Stopes clinics organized a small scale trial of a non-spermicidal diaphragm, they found that it was an ideal form of contraception: 'It didn't require a doctor to fit it, it caused no vaginal infection or cystitis and it was comfortable, it wasn't messy and was easy to get in and out' (Saffron 1984: 15). In fact there was only one significant problem with it – it didn't prevent pregnancy. But when volunteers were told of its alarmingly high failure rate almost half of them refused to give up using it on the grounds that they still felt it was the best contraceptive they had ever tried.

Of course many women do fear unwanted pregnancies and would not wish to use a very unreliable contraceptive method. Yet many women who take 'the pill' admit that they frequently fail to take it 'properly'. Research into the contents of dustbins has found more pill packets with some pills left in them than completely used packets. Doctors appear to be irritated by women's failure to use really effective methods of contraception 'effectively' but, unless young and female themselves, they do not have to remember to go back upstairs and take their pill after an early morning domestic crisis. As we all know, men certainly do not have a particularly good record of using condoms 'effectively'. Yet women who fail to live up to the theoretical efficacy rates of the pill are frequently labelled 'unreliable' and encouraged to use a more long term method. One woman, for example, recalls her doctor recommending the coil 'saying that for me it was probably the only "safe" method as I'm obviously so psychologically and personally unreliable' (Oxford Women's Health Action Group 1984: 8).

However, there is one possible solution to the conflict between safe woman-controlled forms of contraception and the fact that they are in theory less reliable in preventing pregnancy than hormonal contraceptives, IUDs and sterilization. If early abortions were much easier to obtain on the NHS and promoted as a form of contraception rather than a morally dubious last resort, the pill, the IUD and Depo Provera would cease to be so attractive solely on the grounds of efficacy. Most medical textbooks, however, make a clear distinction between contraception and abortion.

Defending the 1967 Abortion Act has always been high on British feminists' agenda. Whilst feminists have had some success in defending women's very limited rights to abortion against several waves of attack from the so-called moral majority, they are still campaigning – unsuccessfully to date – to ensure that all women throughout Britain have access to early NHS abortions. Since 1967, the medical profession in most parts of the country has failed to develop a comprehensive NHS-based abortion service. In 1984 the NHS performed 86 per cent of all abortions in the northern region but only 20 per cent in the West Midlands and only 35 per cent in Yorkshire. Since then, the total percentage of abortions performed on the NHS has declined from 50 to 47 per cent (see Bury 1987). Moreover, women are more likely to experience delays within the NHS than in the private sector. A RCGP/RCOG (1985) study of over 6,000 women undergoing induced abortion found that 27 per cent of women within the NHS had to wait at least three weeks from first consulting their GP to their operation compared to only 14 per cent of women who used the private sector.

Some feminists have hoped that the development of an abortion pill might be the answer to the totally inadequate existing abortion service. In 1988 an abortion pill known as RU486 was licensed in France and promoted as a new, safer, less medicalized form of early termination of pregnancy, on the grounds that it gave women the option of a non-surgical termination which avoided the need for an overnight stay in a hospital or clinic. However, whilst feminists have strongly objected to the anti-abortionists' claim that this drug is equivalent to launching a holocaust against embryos, some feminists have begun to have serious doubts about some of the claims made in relation to RU486. For example, Janice Raymond from the American Institute of Women and Technology has advised British feminists to take a critical look at RU486 (Raymond 1991). She urges them to be wary of this drug on the grounds of safety and side effects as well as the issue of the medical profession's control over it and its users. Behind the myth of do-it-yourself abortion, she argues, lies the fact that 'to maintain safety you require extremely close medical supervision' (Raymond 1991: 35). Moreover, the kind of medical supervision which RU486 requires is not just medical oversight from afar but a highly medicalized treatment regimen which is multi-stepped, time consuming and, for many women, both lengthy and painful. A woman has to ingest the pills at a medical centre, only to return 36 to 48 hours later for either injectable or suppository prostaglandins. Whilst the actual abortion may well take place at home, it may well comprise, according to Raymond 'an excruciating long wait for the fetus to be expelled, often accompanied by pain, bleeding, vomiting, nausea and other complications' (1991: 36). Raymond urges feminists to challenge the medical profession's monopoly over abortion rather than buying into a new type of medically controlled service.

Many doctors express some distaste at being involved in providing an abortion service. Some doctors have strong religious beliefs against all abortions. The 1967 Abortion Act allows doctors and only doctors to determine whether or not a woman's request for an abortion meets the requirements of the Act that her health will be in some way impaired if the pregnancy were to continue. Yet, whilst doctors' complete control over abortion may let politicians off the hook in relation to a complex, controversial 'moral issue', technically a doctor's skills are hardly necessary to perform early abortions. In the Third World, trained paramedics frequently perform safe, early abortions – which is hardly surprising given the fact that abortion by the suction method carried out with only a local anaesthetic is a particularly safe and simple procedure. If trained paramedics can safely perform abortions in one country, why not in another? Why should women wanting early terminations of pregnancies in Britain have to put themselves at the mercy of the medical profession at all? If feminists could achieve the demedicalization of suction abortion, women-centred clinics staffed by predominantly non-medical staff could offer women one stop counselling, terminations and after-termination support. However, given the strength of the anti-abortion lobby in Britain or rather its vociferousness, it is highly unlikely that a feminist campaign to demedicalize the early termination of pregnancy would win any immediate ground on the strength of the logic of its case.

Conclusion

Many women have undoubtedly benefited from the development of modern methods of fertility control. For all their faults and failings, the pill and the IUD have provided very effective protection against unwanted pregnancies for millions of women. The 1967 Abortion Act also has many weaknesses but since its passing women living in Britain no longer die from botched backstreet abortions. However, whilst both the pharmaceutical industry and the medical profession try to persuade women that 'high tech' methods of contraception are both extremely effective and extremely safe, those with no vested interests in these methods have claimed that barrier methods of contraception backed up by demedicalized early abortions would offer safer and more controllable options for fertile women wishing to avoid pregnancy. Yet, while diaphragms and caps are currently available on the NHS – in principle at least to most women who want them – the current system does very little to encourage their use and development. Despite the rise in AIDS and cervical cancer, the medical profession, particularly GPs, continue to advocate the pill and IUDs whilst playing down the efficacy and safety of the cap and diaphragm. These methods are more likely to be readily accessible in family planning clinics which also offer women the chance to see a female doctor. Yet these clinics, far from being promoted by the NHS, are currently under threat (see Godlee 1992). In some areas, family planning clinics have even been closed down, despite the fact that official government policy upholds the principle that women should have a choice of contraceptive services.

The lack of a well-funded easily accessible contraceptive service which would offer all women a genuine and informed choice of contraceptive methods is symptomatic of the current distribution of resources within the new 'competitive' NHS. 'Profitable' high technology branches of medicine based within prestigious trust hospitals continue to attract relatively high levels of funding whilst less prestigious community based services including family planning clinics struggle to survive. Such public parsimony in relation to women's real contraceptive needs can be contrasted with the private market's continued interest in profiting from women as contraceptive consumers. According to Yanoshik and Norsigian, 'oral and injectable contraceptives are amongst the most lucrative of all pharmaceuticals' (1989: 69).

Worldwide, the market for these drugs is worth billions of dollars. Moreover the continuing emphasis within research and development programmes on 'high tech' contraceptive methods ensures their continuing profitability. In the 1980s 60 per cent of research and development (R & D) money for contraception went towards female 'high tech' methods such as oral contraceptives, implants and injectables. Only 3 per cent of R & D funds went on research into female barrier methods, spermicides and natural fertility control methods, and only 7 per cent went toward developing exclusively male forms of contraception (Yanoshik and Norsigian 1989). Figures such as these indicate the main biases which ultimately determine women's experiences of controlling their fertility. Whilst women are the main users of modern forms of contraception, men remain very firmly in control of the development, marketing and distribution of modern contraceptives. This means that women's subjective experiences of using 'high tech' contraception are highly unlikely to form the basis of their future development. Medicalized forms of contraception are not only highly profitable, they also allow population planners to increase their control over women's fertility worldwide. Unfortunately the costs of such programmes are borne disproportionately by women, particularly those women deemed by the population planners to be irresponsible or undesirable reproducers. These women are very rarely fully informed of the risks attached to the long term use of the most 'high tech' forms of contraception.

Understandably some women, particularly those perhaps whose lives are most constrained by either absolute or relative poverty, now actively choose a method of contraception which frees them from the day-to-day decision making and 'hassle' associated with barrier methods of contraception such as the diaphragm. Understandably too, many women do not feel secure or powerful enough to insist that their male partners take more responsibility for preventing conception. Men as a group have proved highly resistant to using any form of contraception which might interfere with their sexual pleasure or desire, whilst women as a group have totally failed to redefine heterosexuality to exclude or even limit penetrative and ejaculatory sex (see, for example, Holland *et al.* 1992). Women's control over their own fertility is thus clearly constrained by forces much wider than those at work within the health care industry.

In recent years the health care industry, following very effective campaigning by women's organizations, has begun to give women more information about the alternative methods of contraception currently available to them. Some doctors have even attempted to treat their female patients as intelligent partners in the search for a method of fertility control which will match their own particular needs and desires, rather than continuing to provide patriarchal and patronizing contraceptive advice. Despite these positive changes, evidence presented in this chapter strongly indicates that the contraceptive services currently available to women in Britain fall a long way short of meeting women's own contraceptive needs and desires. In particular the current developments in the marketing and targeting of implantable hormonal contraceptives should leave women in little doubt that the health care industry intends to continue its control over their fertility. Whilst a perfect form of contraception may prove to be just a feminist pipe dream it is clear that women's own needs are currently taking a rather poor second place to the interests of contraceptive manufacturers, the medical profession, the government and ultimately all sexually active heterosexual men.

2

MATERNITY CARE

Unlike their great grandmothers and grandmothers, pregnant women in Britain today can look forward to a pregnancy and delivery which poses only an extremely small risk to their own lives. In 1918 the maternal mortality rate was 3.79 per 1,000 live births, by 1934 the rate had actually risen to 4.6 per 1,000 but by 1990 the rate was 0.081 per 1,000 maternities (Health Committee 1991: vi). In other words, only eight women now die in childbirth out of every 100,000 women who give birth. The infant mortality rate has also reached an all-time low. In 1900 the infant mortality rate for England and Wales was 154 per thousand births, by 1920 it had dropped to 80 but by 1990 it had fallen to just 8.4 (House of Commons Health Committee 1991: vi). Alongside this dramatic fall in both maternal and infant mortality has gone an equally dramatic change in the place of birth. Before World War I only about 1 per cent of births took place in hospitals, nursing homes and poor law institutions. By 1945 54 per cent of births took place in hospital. By 1990 that figure had risen to approximately 99 per cent (House of Commons Health Committee 1991: vii).

To most obstetricians, the media, health policy makers and many pregnant women themselves, the fact that death rates from childbirth and perinatal mortality rates have fallen dramatically at the same time as hospital births have risen so dramatically is all the proof needed to view the existence of modern antenatal and obstetric care as one of the great success stories of the twentieth century. Newspapers and magazine articles continue to portray the spread of new antenatal screening procedures and expensive obstetric equipment as a great advance for medicine – and of course pregnant women. In August 1987, for example, an article in *The Times* entitled 'Giving birth to the new tech babies' admired Watford General Hospital for having the most advanced maternity unit in Britain. According to one of the three 'energetic' doctors who together had been responsible for the raising of £150,000 of charitable donations to fund the new equipment, the technology now available in units such as this meant that 'there is little excuse for accidents to either mother or child purely as a result of labour. In an ideal unit which we're trying to create we should never have a brain damaged baby' (Tipton cited by Lamb 1987). A woman giving birth in this 'ideal' unit would be continuously connected up to a fetal monitor which would in turn be wired up to a central computer with three TV screens where her progress would be closely observed. This would allow a senior midwife to monitor several patients' progress at once without even having to be in the same room with them (Tipton 1987).

So great has been modern obstetricians' enthusiasm for, and confidence in, their high technology obstetric units, that as a profession they have become ever more reluctant to allow even a tiny minority of 'low risk' women the option of a low tech or natural home birth. One American obstetrician has stated that for him the whole idea of out-of-hospital deliveries 'represents the epitome of "meism"' and that in his opinion, 'out-of-hospital deliveries are the last form of child abuse that is legitimate' (cited in Cohen 1988: 242). Another has argued

> I think the trade-off of being in a modern hospital with all the latest advances available to you versus being in a homelike environment is just no contest. So there are some inconveniences and unpleasantness in being a patient in a hospital. Big deal! The stakes are pretty high and you are only there for a few days. You can damn well bet I wouldn't let my wife or daughter try it.
>
> (cited in Cohen 1988: 246)

British obstetricians tend not to use such colourful language – at least not when speaking on the record – but many of them have expressed very similar viewpoints. For example, a senior representative of the RCOG told the House of Commons Health Committee in 1991

> it would seem to us clear that we feel that the safest place is where the facilities are. The finest facilities will be in the biggest units, fairly good facilities in much smaller units, but these facilities would be better than no facilities at home.
>
> (RCOG 1991: xivii)

Professor Sir Malcolm Macnaughton, past president of the RCOG, wrote in his evidence to the Health Committee

> Women should be confined in hospital as 10 per cent of normal low risk women will require expert treatment in labour and these women cannot

be selected beforehand. Labour can only be said to be normal when it is completed.

(Macnaughton 1991: 816)

Obstetricians not only encourage women to go into hospital for the actual birth, they also run hospital-based antenatal clinics which most women are advised to attend throughout their pregnancy. Women who do not choose to receive medical care and advice from a very early stage in their pregnancy are seen as problematic by maternity staff and have been labelled as 'late attenders' or worse. During the 1980s antenatal care providers put a great deal of effort into researching why some women – particularly poor women and ethnic minority women – failed to use such an obviously beneficial medical service (see, for example, Randhawa 1986). Health care providers then attempted to make antenatal care far more attractive to the deviant minority of late attenders. In some health authorities, for example, crèches were provided by antenatal clinics, in others mobile clinics went out into deprived neighbourhoods (McKee 1984). Behind all this change and activity was the firm belief that much of the 'appalling' gap in infant mortality rates between the social classes and the high infant mortality rates within certain ethnic minorities could be significantly reduced if only women in these groups would use maternity services properly.

Despite the very strong dominant view that antenatal and obstetric care are an essential element of safe pregnancy and childbirth, a vociferous minority of women have remained totally unimpressed by the case for the medicalization of childbirth and have continued to fight for the right to choose low tech forms of maternity care involving home birth.

In this chapter we will critically evaluate obstetricians' claims for the efficacy of high technology maternity care. We will also explore the safety of current medical interventions during pregnancy as well as assessing their impact on pregnant women's emotional well-being. The rise in the practice of fetal medicine will then be briefly analysed before the likely future of maternity care services is discussed.

Antenatal care

Research into pregnant women's satisfaction with antenatal care showed conclusively that during the 1970s and 1980s women strongly disliked the 'cattle market' approach adopted in many hospital-based clinics (see, for example, Mason 1989). Although medical experts agree that one of the key aims of antenatal care should be the giving of advice and reassurance to pregnant women, women themselves have frequently reported that asking for such advice and reassurance in a hospital-based setting is extremely difficult. For example, the National Childbirth Trust (NCT) has cited the findings of research in one consultant clinic which found that 60 per cent of women asked no questions and 50 per cent of women said that they had questions but had felt too intimidated to ask them (NCT 1991: 240). The House of Commons Health Committee also heard evidence that women from ethnic groups where English was not the first language had even greater problems obtaining information from antenatal care staff (House of Commons Health Committee 1991: xviii). Such findings are hardly surprising given research which found, for example, that one-third of all women attending antenatal clinics in one health district never saw the same person twice (AIMS 1991: 466). Research has also shown that doctors working in hospital-based antenatal clinics find the day-to-day worries of their patients at best relatively trivial and boring and at worst ridiculous. Ann Oakley's *Women Confined* (1980) gave a number of examples of doctors treating pregnant women's concerns as a joke. When one woman complained to a doctor that she could not sleep at all because she felt so uncomfortable his only response was 'we need to put you in a hammock don't we?' before he immediately asked her when she had produced her urine sample (Oakley 1980).

According to the National Childbirth Trust comments and complaints from their members have built up a clear picture of

> lack of time at antenatal clinics, failure to explain reasons for procedures and failure to offer information clearly ... many commented that their antenatal care was conducted in an impolite, inconsiderate and offhand way ...
>
> (NCT, 1991: xvi)

Similarly, Sheila Kitzinger reported that

> Even in hospitals which had a delightful atmosphere in the labour suite ... the antenatal clinic often seemed to expectant mothers like a factory in which they were processed through machines, with little personal contact of any kind.
>
> (Kitzinger 1979)

If women find antenatal clinics such an ordeal why do they usually attend dutifully for so many check-ups? Presumably they strongly believe that not to do so might put themselves and their unborn babies at risk. Certainly this is the powerful message given out by the medical profession and health educationists. The Health Education Authority's *Pregnancy Book* advises women, for example 'the earlier you go [for antenatal care] the better. If there is anything wrong, however slight, then it's best to find out early so the problem can be dealt with' (HEA 1991: 27). What most pregnant women are not told, and therefore cannot know, is that there is now a growing body of dissent within the medical and nursing professions which challenges the dominant view that hospital-based antenatal care for all pregnant women plays a major role in reducing perinatal and maternal mortality and morbidity. Indeed some medical experts have now gone so far as to suggest that many of the routine checks performed on all pregnant women during antenatal visits are a waste of time and resources. In September 1993 an editorial in the *British Medical Journal*, for example, argued that the rituals of weighing women in early pregnancy, testing their urine for glucose and listening for a fetal heartbeat were all of little or no value as screening devices (Steer 1993). One leading obstetrician has given up the routine weighing of pregnant women – presumed to be useful in identifying growth retarded babies – on the grounds that it is not, in practice, an accurate predictor of low weight babies (Siddle in Howarth 1991: 57). Not only is this procedure now questioned as an accurate diagnostic tool there is also evidence that, despite it being an extremely simple and non-invasive test, it may unnecessarily cause some women acute stress. If a woman is identified during routine antenatal care as failing to put on enough weight the consequences for her may be quite extreme. One woman, for example, has reported, 'I dreaded going to the clinic because I knew they would go on about my weight'. When this woman reached her estimated delivery date she was offered an elective Caesarean but gave birth to a very normal 6lb 4oz daughter. She commented, 'I really didn't mind about the Caesarean. By that time I was so terrified that my baby wasn't getting enough food and so miserable that I just wanted the pregnancy to be over (Howarth, 1991: 57). Even if routine weighing does sometimes detect a failure to put on weight, research carried out in the Oxford region has suggested that this is not necessarily an indication that the baby is at risk, since the researchers found that nearly half a large sample of pregnant women failed to put on weight in the last trimester without adverse effects (Howarth 1991).

Whilst some of the routine simple tests carried out on millions of pregnant women may be less safe and efficacious than was once thought, most attention in recent years has focused on the newer so-called 'high tech' screening procedures such as ultrasound, amniocentesis and chorion villus sampling (CVS).

Ultrasound was first developed during World War II to track down enemy submarines. Medical ultrasound scanning began to be used as a diagnostic aid in high risk pregnancies during the 1970s but by the late 1980s it was routinely used in most antenatal clinics. Most obstetricians are absolutely convinced that ultrasound is a perfectly safe procedure which, in expert hands, can provide a whole range of useful information from determining the exact age of the fetus to checking for multiple births and fetal position and to indicating some types of fetal abnormalities. The official line from the RCOG is that the wave intensity currently used in routine scans is 'probably safe' (McTaggart 1990), whilst pregnant women who ask about the safety of ultrasound are usually reassured that the procedure is 'as safe as TV'. A number of critics of ultrasound on the other hand have expressed a range of concerns over its ever increasing use in routine antenatal care. According to its critics, ultrasound scanning is a major form of medical experimentation which has never been subjected to the type of clinical trials which would be necessary to rule out any long term harmful effects of its widescale use. The Association for Improvements in Maternity Service (AIMS), for example, 'strongly question the ethics of exposing the majority of children born in this country to a potentially dangerous procedure whose long term effects have not been adequately researched' (1991: 486).

A few research scientists have claimed that ultrasound does have a subtle but possibly significant effect on body cells (see Bolsen 1982). One study purported to demonstrate higher rates of left handedness among children who had been exposed to ultrasound in the womb (Salvesen 1993). In 1993 a report in *The Lancet* of the Perth randomized controlled trial of frequent prenatal ultrasound examinations concluded that frequent ultrasound scans appeared to be associated with low birthweight and concluded 'it is ... plausible that frequent exposure to ultrasound may have influenced fetal growth' (Newnham *et al.* 1993: 887). In the United States various official bodies have insisted that ultrasound should not be used routinely on pregnant women. In 1984, for example, a panel of American experts concluded that 'the data do not allow a recommendation for routine screening at this time' (Butler 1984) yet that is exactly what is occurring throughout Britain.

Whilst any possible long term risks associated with routine ultrasound testing remain at present very largely hypothetical, the more immediate risks of ultrasound are well proven. For example, the risk of ultrasound falsely detecting some type of fetal abnormality is a very real one. One study from Harvard showed that among 3,100 scans, 18 babies were erroneously picked out as abnormal (McTaggart 1990). In the most extreme cases such misdiagnoses by ultrasound can lead to a pregnant woman opting to abort an apparently abnormal foetus which proves to have been perfectly normal. AIMS gave evidence to the House of Commons Health Committee stating that they knew of a number of cases where this had happened (AIMS 1991: 486). Even when a mistake made by an ultrasound operator, not all of whom are highly trained or skilled in the use of this technology, is later detected before any drastic action has been taken, the woman concerned will have undoubtedly suffered very high levels of anxiety and distress.

If routine ultrasound scanning clearly carries some risk of wrong diagnosis and concomitant anxiety and distress to the pregnant woman thus tested, are such costs nevertheless outweighed by the benefits it brings? They are not, according to the American College of Obstetrics and Gynaecology in 1984, which stated 'no well-controlled study' had yet 'proved that routine screening of prenatal patients will improve the outcome of pregnancy' (McTaggart 1990: 2). In 1993 the authors of a meta-analysis of randomized trials evaluating the effect of routine ultrasound scanning involving 15,935 pregnancies concluded

> Routine ultrasound scanning does not improve the outcome of pregnancy in terms of an increased number of live births or of reduced perinatal mortality. Routine ultrasound scanning may be effective and useful as a

screening for malformation. Its use for this purpose, however, should be made explicit and take into account the risk of false positive diagnosis in addition to ethical issues.

(Bucher and Schmidt 1993)

Despite very negative research findings such as this, most doctors continue to use ultrasound routinely during antenatal care and continue to place more faith in the results of these machines than in the knowledge of pregnant women themselves – sometimes with tragic results. AIMS has reported several cases where women who have been sure of the date of conception have been told that ultrasound testing proved them wrong. Their babies were then induced on the grounds that the doctors 'knew' that the pregnancy had gone beyond term but then premature babies were in fact delivered and in some cases died. Conversely, in one case reported to AIMS, medical staff again did not believe the woman's own dates but relied on an ultrasound reading showing a much later than expected date of delivery. When she went into labour she was given drugs to suppress what the medical staff believed to be a premature labour but in the event a full-term fetus was delivered dead (AIMS 1991: 486).

Not only has the ever-increasing use of ultrasound contributed to the tendency of the medical profession to downgrade or ignore women's own knowledge of their pregnancy, it has also played a role in diminishing the traditional knowledge and skills of midwives. In 1991 midwifery delegates from all over the UK attended a seminar in London (funded by a supplier of ultrasound equipment) designed to encourage them 'to seize the opportunity' to learn how to use ultrasound as a routine part of their work (Cunningham 1992). In future, if the manufacturers of ultrasound machines have their way, health care providers may increasingly become incapable of detecting potential complications of pregnancy by straightforward physical examinations.

One of the unstated advantages of the spread of ultrasound scanning is that doctors and other health care providers find the equipment interesting and exciting to use. Such equipment also plays a role in maintaining the prestige of this branch of modern medicine. The spread of ultrasound machines throughout the hospitals of Britain has certainly been a boon to the manufacturers of such equipment but much less of a boon to district health authorities struggling to provide comprehensive health care services during a time of severe resource constraints. Given the mounting research evidence on the inefficacy of the routine ultrasound scanning of all pregnant women, one might venture to suggest that district health authorities should look very closely at their expenditure on these machines and their running cost and at the very least attempt to restrict their routine use and confine their availability to just a few specialist centres. Unfortunately, rational and logical use of health care resources rarely coincides with politically popular priorities and no doubt any attempt to restrict the use of ultrasound during pregnancy would attract a media response that women's and babies' lives were being jeopardized by funding cuts.

Whilst virtually all pregnant women are now given at least one routine ultrasound scan, amniocentesis, a test used to detect Down's Syndrome and some other fetal abnormalities such as spina bifida, is not routinely given to all pregnant women but is now usually offered to all women over the age of 35 or 40. The procedure involves putting a needle through the woman's abdomen into the amniotic sac and removing some amniotic fluid for testing. Given under local anaesthetic, the procedure is usually more uncomfortable than painful but it clearly creates some anxiety in many of those who undergo it. According to *The New Our Bodies, Ourselves*

> Whilst some women find the procedure easy, others find it an unpleasant, upsetting experience. Most women agree that it is wise to rest afterwards for at least a day as you may well feel quite shaky and shocked.
>
> (Phillips and Rakusen 1989: 371)

One woman has described how when she went for amniocentesis

> The doctor couldn't get the needle in the right place and kept moving it around for a long time. This really hurt and I was upset and anxious. Finally he took the needle out and tried again. The second time there was no problem but I was quite distraught by that time.
>
> (Phillips and Rakusen 1989: 371)

Amniocentesis cannot be performed until the sixteenth week of pregnancy and the results for Down's Syndrome take approximately two to three weeks to come through. If an abnormality is detected modern medicine cannot offer to put it right but only to terminate the pregnancy. This means that a woman whose test proves positive has to make the very difficult decision of whether to go through a very late abortion or to give birth to a 'handicapped' child without knowing the degree of handicap that child will suffer. Women who have personally faced this choice have described how traumatic it can be. One woman who underwent an abortion after a positive amniocentesis result has commented

> Doctors must understand the consequences of offering tests. The some-times all-too-glib 'Oh you're 40 we can test to see if the baby is abnormal' can mean that a woman has to reject her wanted child. We, as women, must be aware that prior knowledge of our baby's ill health might be knowledge we would rather not have.
>
> (Statham, 1987)

Not only is a positive amniocentesis test result a mixed benefit to those women who receive it but amniocentesis testing is by no means risk free, which is why it is mainly restricted to older women who are deemed to be at much higher risk of giving birth to a handicapped child. In the mid-1970s a large scale controlled study undertaken in England and Wales found that, even in the hands of skilled specialists, the amniocentesis procedure killed 1.5 per cent of the fetuses tested. In other words, over one woman in every hundred undergoing this test could lose her unborn child as a direct result of it, although a more recent estimate of the risk of miscarriage has put it at between 1.5 and only 0.2 per cent (McNay *et al.* 1984: 411).

In the late 1980s the popular press hailed a new test, chorion villus sampling (CVS) for Down's Syndrome, as the potential answer to every older pregnant woman's prayer. This new test can be given between the ninth and twelfth week of pregnancy and thus enable women to have a much earlier abortion should the test prove positive. Unfortunately, a large Medical Research Council (MRC) funded study of 3,000 women found that those given the CVS test were even more likely to miscarry than those undergoing amniocentesis, and the risk of losing a baby through CVS has been calculated as approximately 5 per cent (McTaggart 1991). The study also found one definite and two possible false positives in the CVS group and one false negative. There have also been reports of limb abnormalities of babies whose mothers underwent CVS (Firth *et al.* 1991). The initial enthusiasm for this new test now seems somewhat premature but meanwhile another new test, serum screening, is now being increasingly used instead of maternal age in order to assess women at risk of giving birth to a Down's Syndrome baby (Statham and Green 1993). Whilst this test is in itself non-invasive, it may well be given to mostly younger women on the grounds that it is harmless and thus lead to more women being referred for the far from 'perfectly safe' amniocentesis test in order to confirm the serum test finding. A recent study of women's experiences of this new serum test found that even after receipt of negative amniocentesis tests following a positive serum screening result some women remained anxious that there was something wrong with their baby (Statham and Green 1993).

Whilst most older women appear to welcome amniocentesis and other such tests on the grounds that the usual negative result is reassuring, a few women have argued strongly that before women accept these tests they should think very carefully about the implications for themselves, should the test prove positive, and also about the wider implications of the use of these tests. One 40-year-old Canadian woman, for example, has written about how she 'instinctively rejected' what she saw as 'another medical invasion of women's bodies' but then found herself thinking more and more about the 'wider social implication of amniocentesis'. 'As individuals' she has argued

> we might decide, understandably enough that we don't want or can't cope with the demands of raising a child with physical or mental disabilities. Collectively, however, these choices add up to something more chilling: a wholesale societal rejection of disabled people, a kind of reproductive 'quality control'.
>
> (McDonnell 1988: 23)

From this perspective, far from giving older women more control over their pregnancy, amniocentesis can be seen as part of a much wider programme which will eventually give scientists and the medical profession far more control over the whole reproductive process and even the creation of life itself.

Intervention in childbirth

Whilst public debates over the efficacy and safety of antenatal screening procedures are relatively recent, controversy over the medicalization of childbirth itself has raged for several decades. Critics of modern obstetric practice have consistently complained that a whole range of medical interventions during childbirth are both ineffectual and also physically and psychologically harmful to women on the receiving end of them. In response to these critics, some routine procedures are now less commonly used in British maternity units. During the 1970s, for example, many women going into hospital to give birth were routinely 'prepped' or shaved and given an enema, procedures which many women understandably found degrading and unpleasant. Critics then proved that these routines fulfilled no useful medical purpose and that if anything they actually increased the risk of infection to both mother and child. In response many obstetric units have now dropped both procedures although they cannot yet be assumed to be totally abandoned (see Phillips and Rakusen 1989: 390).

Another cause of discontent and concern amongst pregnant women throughout the 1970s was the widespread use of the drug oxytocin to induce and speed up the labour process. In her national survey of induction in the mid-1970s Ann Cartwright found that nearly half the consultant obstetricians she interviewed said that inductions had increased their job satisfaction because 'it had enabled more planning of deliveries, tidier departments and happier mothers' (Cartwright cited by Oakley 1993: 33). Doctors apparently also believed that women would appreciate the much shorter labours which could be achieved using 'active management' techniques such as induction by oxytocin. Many women themselves, however, found the strong contractions which usually followed such inductions difficult to bear without painkillers (NCT 1975). Moreover, researchers found during the 1970s that inductions could lead not only to increased use of painkillers during labour but also to an increase in episiotomies, forceps deliveries and even Caesarean sections (Kitzinger 1979). Such research findings and the anger of women who believed that some inductions were being carried out not for medical reasons but because medical staff did not wish to work over a weekend or through the night, led eventually to a decline in the percentage of labours induced by oxytocin. After rising dramatically from under 10 per cent of deliveries in the early 1960s to a national peak of almost 40 per cent in the early 1970s, the induction rate then declined steadily to about 12 per cent in 1988–89 (House of

GRIMSBY COLLEGE LIBRARY

Commons Health Committee 1991: p x/ix). This does not mean, however, that active management of births is now any less active in many hospitals. For example, a postal survey carried out for the NCT in the late 1980s found that of the 3,000 women who sent back their questionnaires over 50 per cent had their membranes artificially ruptured (ARM) which is an alternative method of speeding up the labour process. Fifty-seven per cent of women who had delivered in consultant units had ARM compared to only 28 per cent of the 168 women who had given birth at home. In some cases women reported that hospital staff had performed ARM without any warning. One woman wrote

> While being examined the midwife said 'I'll just break your waters' – instrument at the ready. I said 'Oh no please don't'. She said it would make it quicker for me. I was horrified – all I wanted was for my labour to take its course naturally.
>
> (NCT 1989: 29)

Some mothers told the NCT researchers that they felt ARM had been beneficial for them because it had speeded up a slow labour. Others, however, complained about the pain which followed ARM. The NCT researchers concluded that 'like induction in the 1970s ARM may have become increasingly common without any proper evaluation of its effects on the mother, her labour and her baby' (NCT 1989: 56).

One reason given to women by hospital staff for performing ARM was the need to carry out 'accurate monitoring' via scalp electrode. Electronic fetal monitoring (EFM) was unusual and experimental in the early 1970s but two decades later it has become almost routine for most consultant units. One postal survey of 276 consultants recently found that the number of monitoring machines in use in their units almost doubled between 1977 and 1984 (Wheble et al. 1989). Doctors have claimed that the increased use of these sophisticated and expensive machines will reduce the risk of brain damage from fetal distress and that, in particular, it will prevent unnecessary cases of cerebral palsy. In 1975, for example, two American obstetricians suggested that fetal heart rate monitoring during labour could 'reduce perinatal mortality and morbidity by 50%'. They went on to talk about reducing the number of mentally handicapped infants by half and claimed that the huge financial savings made by the avoidance and prevention of mental retardation would far outstrip a projected annual cost of total intrapartum monitoring in the USA of $100 million per year (Quilligan and Paul 1975). Fourteen years later, however, an editorial in The Lancet argued that whilst the immoderate and unfounded claims of the early proponents of electronic fetal monitoring might be excused, obstetricians and paediatricians no longer had any excuse for continuing to make totally unsubstantiated claims for such monitoring. The editorial concluded that 'the vast majority of cases of cerebral palsy are exceedingly unlikely to be preventable by more intensive forms of intrapartum care' and that 'the continued willingness of doctors to reinforce the fable that intrapartum care is an important determinant of cerebral palsy can only be regarded as shooting the speciality of obstetrics in the foot' (*The Lancet*, 1989: 1252).

Cerebral palsy is not the only problem which electronic fetal monitoring has patently failed to solve. In 1987 an article in *The Lancet* reviewed the results of eight prospective randomized controlled trials of such monitoring. The article concluded that none of these trials had suggested 'any major advantage of EFM over intermittent surveillance in terms of neonatal mortality or morbidity' (Prentice and Lind 1987: 1375).

Whilst enthusiastic supporters of EFM have notably failed to provide any clear evidence of benefits from its ever-increasing use, research has demonstrated a number of significant costs. Firstly, EFM increases the Caesarean section rate as it leads to a high rate of detection of apparent fetal distress. One study reported that 71 to 95 per cent of babies delivered operatively for presumed fetal distress were not actually found to be clinically distressed at birth (Billingsley 1987). Women themselves on the other hand have undoubtedly been distressed during EFM. Women have reported increased discomfort caused partly by being attached to the monitoring equipment and partly by being less able to move about whilst being monitored (AIMS 1991: 484). Women have also reported medical staff appearing to be far more interested in the monitoring machines than in the woman herself (AIMS 1991: 484). There is also anecdotal evidence of machines which keep breaking down or being unreliable. According to AIMS, one husband was so disturbed by his belief that something awful had happened when the monitor stopped recording whilst he was on his own with his wife that he arranged to have a vasectomy immediately after the birth (AIMS 1991: 484). Women subjected to EFM not only risk physical discomfort and emotional stress, they and their babies also run a much greater risk of infection from the use of internal fetal monitors. In one study 85 per cent of babies suffered a post delivery rash after having an electrode attached to their scalp whilst in the womb, whilst 20 per cent suffered from scalp abscess (Phillips and Rakusen 1989).

Despite mounting evidence of side effects from EFM and total lack of firm evidence of any major benefits of its increasingly routine use EFM has now become an accepted technology that is an unquestioned part of every health authority's budget. As AIMS has commented, one wonders how much more evidence of its ineffectiveness and harmful side effects will need to be accumulated before health policy makers take a stand against EFM's ever widening use.

Critics of interventionist obstetric procedures such as induction and electronic fetal monitoring claim that not only do such procedures do more harm than good when evaluated individually but also that use of such procedures during early labour greatly increases the likelihood of surgical intervention at a later stage. Certainly the incidence of Caesarean section has risen dramatically over the last two decades. The most dramatic increase has taken place in the USA where by the mid-1980s the national Caesarean section rate was as high as 24 per cent. In Britain the national rate is much lower – at around 13 per cent in 1992 – but that is still nearly three times the rate of 4.9 per cent recorded in 1970 (Treffers and Pel 1993). Moreover, according to the NCT, official national figures probably underestimate the actual rate of Caesarean section. One research study found that in 1985 over a fifth of maternity units had a Caesarean rate of 14 per cent or over (Francome 1989: 11).

In 1983 the Maternity Alliance undertook a survey of Caesarean sections in which 135 obstetricians were asked to explain the rising rate. Their most common explanation (41 per cent) was the change in treatment of breech deliveries, as many maternity units have moved towards 100 per cent Caesarean section for breech presentation. Twenty-eight per cent of respondents mentioned fear of litigation as a significant factor in their choice of Caesarean deliveries. One doctor commented

> should I produce a brain-damaged baby by a forceps delivery in 1983, that child can accuse me of negligence in a court of law until 2004 ... I like to think it does not unduly influence my clinical judgement.
>
> (Francome 1986: 101)

A third reason given for the rise, by 25 per cent of respondents, was the growth in fetal monitoring. In 1990 a study reported in *The Lancet* found that a detailed audit of 50 Caesarean operations carried out for fetal distress showed that in 30 per cent of cases at least four of five assessors conducting a clinical audit of the cases disagreed with the decision to carry out immediate Caesarean section. The study concluded that one-third of Caesarean operations carried out on the grounds of fetal distress may be unnecessary (Barrett *et al.* 1990: 549).

One reason why doctors now perform so many Caesarean operations is that they are relatively so much safer than in past decades. Nevertheless, the risk of maternal death, although very low is significantly higher for Caesareans than for vaginal deliveries. Women undergoing a Caesarean also face relatively high risks of post-operative morbidity. One large study undertaken in the early 1980s found that 17 per cent of women suffered from wound inflammation whilst 1 per cent suffered major sepsis (Macfarlane and Mugford 1986: 6). Women not only run a high risk of physical problems after a Caesarean, there is also growing evidence of emotional problems and distress following this major surgical procedure. One American researcher found that

> women who had been delivered by Cesarean were significantly more negative about their birth experience ... experienced more serious and long lasting depression and did not 'feel like a mother' (a measure of attachment and bonding) till much later than vaginally delivered women.
>
> (Doering, 1979 cited in Brackbill *et al.* 1984: 26)

A recent British study found that women who delivered by Caesarian section took significantly longer than those delivered vaginally to feel close to their infants and these differences persisted for several months after the birth (Hillan 1992: 163).

Critics of the rising use of Caesareans do not deny that they can sometimes be a life saving operation, for example if a woman is suffering from severe pre-eclampsia or if the umbilical cord has prolapsed. Doctors who defend the rise in Caesarean sections have claimed, however, that they produce a 'superior outcome' for many babies (Brackbill *et al.* 1984). Yet there is no clear statistical evidence to link a rise in Caesarean sections to any fall in perinatal mortality or morbidity. One study at the National Maternity Hospital in Dublin found that perinatal mortality in Dublin fell significantly between 1965 and 1980 despite no increase in the Caesarean rate. The report concluded 'these results do not support the contention that the expansion in Caesarean birth rates has contributed significantly to reduced perinatal mortality rates in recent years' (Phillips and Rakusen 1989: 395). More radical critics go further to suggest that far from contributing to a lowering of perinatal mortality and morbidity, the rising tide of Caesarean sections along with other forms of obstetric interventions has actually contributed to perinatal mortality and morbidity. Marjorie Tew, for example, has claimed that 'the years when hospitalization [of childbirth] increased most were the years when perinatal mortality declined least. There is a strong negative correlation between these figures' (Tew 1991: ix).

Tew is one of the few critics of obstetric intervention who does not accept that it is at least of great benefit to the minority of pregnant women who fall into the genuinely 'high risk' category. Tew claims that

> far from supporting the assumption that obstetric management is especially advantageous for births at high risk the results manifestly discredit this basic principle on which the justification of obstetric management relies.
>
> (1991: 587)

Tew points out that when things go wrong in labour and appear to necessitate emergency 'high tech' intervention they often do so because of previous medical interventions which have directly caused harm to the mother and/or child. For example, pain relieving drugs often given during artificially induced labours are known sometimes to cause breathing difficulties in newborn babies which may necessitate their instant transfer to a neonatal intensive care unit. Obstetricians may then argue that birth is a highly risky business and all mothers should give birth as close as possible to such life saving facilities as neonatal intensive care units.

Changing childbirth?

In 1992 the House of Commons Health Committee published its report *Maternity Services* in which it vigorously challenged the dominant view that a high technology hospital-based maternity service was essential to ensure the well-being of all pregnant women and their babies. The Committee concluded that

> the present imposition of a rigid pattern of frequent antenatal visits is not grounded in any good scientific base and . . . there is no evidence that such a pattern is medically necessary . . . Hospitals are not the appropriate place to care for healthy women.
>
> (House of Commons Health Committee 1991: xliii)

It also stated 'on the basis of what we have heard, this committee must draw the conclusion that the policy of encouraging all women to give birth in hospitals cannot be justified on the grounds of safety' (House of Commons Health Committee 1991: xii). Jean Robinson of the Association for the Improvement of Maternity Services has said that she wept on reading this report because 'at last somebody has listened and believed us . . . obstetricians wouldn't listen. We were really thought of as cranks' (Robinson, in Dobson 1992).

In response to the Select Committee's report the government set up an expert committee 'to review policy on NHS maternity care, particularly during childbirth, and to make recommendations'. This Expert Maternity Group, as it became known, completed its work rather appropriately in nine months. Its report *Changing Childbirth* reinforced the Select Committee's emphasis on women's right to choose the kind of medical care they wanted. It also argued that

> the issue of safety . . . used as an overriding principle, may become an excuse for unnecessary intervention and technological surveillance which detract from the experience of the mother . . . safety is not an absolute concept. It is part of a greater picture encompassing all aspects of health and well being. Each woman should be approached as an individual and given clear and unbiased information on the options that are available to her.
>
> (Expert Maternity Group 1993: 9)

The conclusions of this 'woman centred' report were in marked contrast to previous government reports on maternity care which had accepted without question obstetricians' claims that high technology hospital-based care was essential to ensure the safety of all mothers and babies. *Changing Childbirth* recommended that within five years every pregnant woman should know one midwife who would ensure continuity of care, and that at least 30 per cent of women should have a midwife as 'the lead professional' throughout their pregnancy and should be admitted to a maternity unit under the management of a midwife rather than a consultant obstetrician. The report also recommended that antenatal care should be provided 'in the community' wherever possible, that a thorough review of routine antenatal check-ups should be carried out and that routine antenatal visits for women with uncomplicated pregnancies – apart from the first – should be halved from around 12 to six. The Expert Maternity Group believed that such radical changes in maternity care could well occur within five years given the existence of 'a new spirit abroad in maternity services which can be harnessed to bring about change' (Expert Maternity Group 1993: 71). Certainly the radical recommendations of this group were in themselves a major shift by health policy makers away from the ever-increasing medicalization and hospitalization of all pregnant women. Moreover, many midwives and at least some obstetricians will welcome this change of emphasis and support any moves actually to implement it. However, before concluding that most pregnant women in Britain will soon experience a very different type of maternity care, we should pause to consider a number of serious obstacles to such radical changes. First, policy makers still give a leading role to obstetricians in the care of all women 'when the pregnancy is more complicated' (Expert Maternity Group 1993: 6). A key problem with this apparently logical recommendation is the way in which obstetricians determine whether or not a pregnancy is 'complicated' or 'high risk'.

Obstetricians are totally dependent on a supply of pregnant women as patients. They also need to be generally regarded as having unique and superior knowledge and skills in relation to pregnancy and childbirth in order to continue to enjoy the high status (and high material rewards) currently awarded to them by our society. A growing number of leading obstetricians are now conceding that community-based maternity service may well be more appropriate than hospital-based care for 'low risk' women. It is quite possible, therefore, that within the foreseeable future more pregnant women will be 'allowed', if they so wish, to give birth either in a midwife controlled hospital unit or even at home. This would be particularly welcomed by those women who have experienced extreme antagonism and resistance from their doctors and/or local health authority staff when they have attempted to have a home birth. According to AIMS at least three women 'have been threatened with enforced hospitalisation under the Mental Health Act when they asked for a home birth' (1991: 478). However even if the Expert Maternity Group's most optimistic expectations are fulfilled it is clear that only women defined by the medical profession as 'low risk' will be 'allowed' to opt for a home birth. Obstetricians will certainly continue to insist that all 'high risk' women should give birth under their care and that their labour and deliveries should continue to be 'actively managed' using the latest high tech equipment and procedures. They may also continue to define high proportions of pregnant women as at 'high risk'. In one 1989 study in West Berkshire, for example, only 30 per cent of all births were judged as 'low risk' enough not to need obstetric management (see Tew 1991: 584). According to Marjorie Tew the concept of low and high risk in relation to pregnant women is highly subjective and actually serves to promote the professional interests of obstetricians rather than the well-being of women and babies themselves (1991: 588). Tew's claim receives some support from one study of antenatal clinics at a London teaching hospital which found that the consultant chose to see doctors' wives, lawyers' wives and other higher income group women. The senior registrar would then choose to see the next socioeconomic group leaving women in lower income groups who are most at risk of complications during pregnancy to be seen by the most junior doctors (Arnold 1985).

Tew claims that the criteria currently used by obstetricians to define risk are found, on analysis, to be very unreliable predictions of outcome and that only in a small minority of cases is the high risk predicted actually realized. If one accepts Tew's claim, any move towards community-based low tech antenatal care could still leave many pregnant women in the 'high risk' category who would still find it very difficult to avoid being drawn into consultant-based maternity care and concomitant highly medicalized screening programmes. Moreover, even women who would be deemed 'low risk' enough to avoid hospital-based antenatal care during most of their pregnancy might well still attend a hospital clinic for at least one routine visit and would be highly unlikely to avoid the now ubiquitous ultrasound scanning. Indeed, one midwife who advocates a community-based system suggested to the House of Commons Health Committee

> the obstetric team might screen all pregnant women once, possibly at 20 weeks, when the results of screening including ultrasound anomalies scan and AFP results are available. This could give obstetricians and women of normal pregnancies confidence that the correct type of management had been agreed.
>
> (House of Commons Health Committee 1991: xliv)

Another growing threat to any attempt to demedicalize pregnancy and childbirth is the growth of fetal medicine in which doctors treat the fetus as a patient in its own right. Rather than retreating from a policy of fetal screening which critics claim produces fewer benefits and far more costs than most doctors acknowledge, medical researchers and obstetricians continue to develop new, more exciting forms of fetal screening. For example, the technique of 'fetoscopy' involves inserting a minute lens through the abdomen wall into the womb. The lens can then be replaced by a needle with which to take samples. This new technique allows specialists to undertake new forms of fetal examination and even to perform surgery on the fetus whilst it is still in the womb (see Phillips and Rakusen 1989: 371). Whilst specialists are understandably excited by the new range of surgical possibilities opened up by fetoscopy, its growing use raises serious problems for women, since not only will fetoscopy increase the medicalization of many pregnancies, it also raises the danger of women being forced to undergo medical procedures against their wishes for the sake of the fetus.

In 1987 a 27-year-old American woman who was six months pregnant and terminally ill with cancer wanted to continue her pregnancy until at least

28 weeks when her baby would have a better chance of survival. The hospital, however, ignored the wishes of the patient, her husband and her parents and obtained a court order for an immediate Caesarean section. The baby did not survive the operation and the woman died two days later (Shearer 1989). A higher court later reversed the earlier legal decision after the case attracted a great deal of media attention, possibly because the woman concerned was white and middle-class, but it was by no means a unique case. In 1986 an American survey reported 21 attempts by hospital specialists to obtain court orders to force obstetrical interventions on pregnant women, 15 of which were for Caesarean section (Kolder *et al.* 1987). Ironically, US law would not force an American mother to undergo surgery for the sake of a child once it had been born (for example, she would not be forced to donate a kidney if her child had kidney disease), yet many American obstetricians appear quite happy to deny pregnant women similar rights. Four American obstetricians argued in 1979, for example, that

> if the child is capable of being born alive and the patient does not consent to being subjected to a given treatment directed to save the fetus, the doctor must be legally entitled to warn the patient that she is committing a felony.
>
> (Leiberman *et al.* 1979: 515)

In 1985 46 per cent of leading American specialists in one survey believed that mothers who were thought to be endangering their unborn baby by refusing medical advice should be forcibly detained in hospital and 47 per cent thought other procedures beside Caesareans should be enforced by court order. Only 25 per cent of those surveyed consistently upheld a mentally competent woman's right to refuse medical advice (Shearer 1989). In Britain, apart from one isolated case, judges have resisted giving the fetus any legal rights and have argued that an unborn child has 'no existence independent of its mother'. However, given the extent to which Britain tends to follow American trends in health care, albeit in a far less dramatic way, British women should not assume that the dangers posed to them by the growth of 'fetal rights' and fetal medicine are still far distant. A survey of British obstetricians carried out in 1986 and 1987 found that developments in neonatal intensive care – which had dramatically improved the outcome of very premature babies – had been responsible for an increase in early Caesarean sections (Francome 1989). The fact that babies born as early as 26 weeks can now survive due to intensive neonatal care is clearly increasing the pressure on obstetricians to treat the fetus as a patient in its own right. The danger is that doctors who have traditionally put 'safety' above other considerations, such as women's experiences of childbirth, will adopt the concept of fetal rights as a weapon in the war for control over the childbirth process. The history of the rising power of obstetricians over the birthing process strongly suggests that women's rights to control their own bodies may yet again be about to face a powerful challenge.

Most of the American women forced to undergo medical procedures against their express wishes for the sake of a fetus were poor women of colour. Affluent white women are more likely to be able to avoid the worst forms of medicalized childbirth. In Britain, for example, a small minority of articulate wealthy women already buy the type of maternity care they prefer. If the NHS cannot provide them with the type of birth they desire, affluent women can now employ an 'independent' midwife and have a privatized natural home birth. Alternatively, women for whom money is no object can opt to give birth in private clinics which specialize in providing women with 'ideal' birthing environments. One woman, for example, whose NHS consultant insisted that a natural birth could not be countenanced as her baby was in a breech position, decided to take the very expensive option of attending a private clinic in London where she gave birth 'naturally' and found the whole experience to be 'magical' (Francis 1986: 21).

In the late nineteenth century all women who could afford to do so gave birth at home. Only women too poor to have any alternative reluctantly went into public institutions, including the great voluntary hospitals, to give birth. Their reluctance was understandable given the horrendously high maternal mortality rates in hospitals at that time. In the late twentieth century a hospital birth is undoubtedly extremely safe for mothers and babies but according to radical critics it may well be less safe, particularly in terms of maternal morbidity, than community-based alternatives. Since hospital-based obstetricians are unlikely to give up their empires voluntarily and since an under-funded NHS is equally unlikely to be able to provide the highest levels of personal care and attention now demanded by its more affluent 'consumers', we may well see in the not too distant future a return, albeit on a small scale, to a traditional class split within maternity care. Middle and upper class women may increasingly exercise the privilege of the true market place and opt out of the NHS into alternative private maternity care services designed to give them the type of birth they desire in the place of their choice. Meanwhile, poor women will continue to go into financially perilous NHS hospitals to give birth with less and less personal care and attention as the costs of the service, apart from the high technology insisted upon by obstetricians, are pared to the bone. These women will probably continue to assume that the discomforts they endure are a price well worth paying for the increased safety offered by modern obstetrical practices.

Unfortunately, much of the evidence presented in this chapter suggests that this faith in modern obstetrics is unjustified. For many pregnant women, including some of those in the so-called 'high risk' group, the costs of modern maternity care probably outweigh the benefits and this equation is unlikely to change significantly even if the providers of maternity care do eventually succumb to the growing pressures on them to shift towards a much more user-friendly service.

3

INFERTILITY TREATMENT

During the 1970s and 1980s medical treatment for patients with infertility problems was transformed from a low status medical backwater with very little to offer to a highly prestigious specialty at the cutting edge of medical research and technology. In Britain the new reproductive technologies such as in vitro fertilization (IVF) and gamete intra fallopian tube transfer (GIFT) are now widely available in the private health care sector but are still strictly rationed within the NHS. At first sight the rapid development of these new technologies appears to have given women a whole new range of reproductive choices. Women with blocked fallopian tubes can now be assisted to conceive. Women without eggs of their own can carry and bear their partner's genetic offspring by using eggs donated by another woman. Even post-menopausal women can now be assisted to become 'mothers' using donated eggs. Babies conceived with the help of infertility specialists were originally hailed by the popular press as 'miracle' babies and many women who have finally conceived a child of their own with the help of reproductive technology have nothing but praise for the specialists who made 'their dream come true'. Why then should a growing number of feminists regard these new technologies and those who control them as a major threat to all women's reproductive freedom? Why have feminists who fought long and hard for women's access to medical forms of contraception and abortion decided to fight against the continuing expansion of reproductive technologies which, their promoters claim, simply expand women's control over their reproductive lives? In this chapter we will first outline the claims made for the new reproductive technologies. We will then evaluate these techniques in terms of their efficacy, their safety and their potential impact on women's reproductive rights, before concluding by questioning whether women as a whole have benefited from the creation of a whole new field of medical science.

The case for new reproductive technologies

Those who advocate the development and expansion of new reproductive technologies such as IVF and GIFT portray their development – at least when talking to the media – as primarily a humane response to the desperate needs of infertile individuals or couples. Infertility is conceptualized as an illness or disease, the new reproductive technologies are then represented as a miracle cure. For example, the well known British infertility specialist Robert Winston told *The Observer*, 'Infertility is actually a terrible disease affecting our sexuality and well being' (Winston 1985). Those pleading for extra public funding of the IVF/GIFT programmes have told the media that they are being 'besieged' by childless women 'begging for help'.

An American infertility specialist has claimed, 'The number of couples seeking medical help for infertility is increasing dramatically' partly because of a trend towards delayed childbearing and partly because of 'the rapidly diminishing availability of adoptable infants'. 'Intense pressure' is therefore being exerted on the health care system to provide effective infertility therapy to couples 'willing to pursue almost any reasonable effort toward achieving their goal of parenthood' (Haney 1987: 543). One British infertility specialist has even argued that infertility treatment should have one of the highest priorities within the NHS and 'should come before chemotherapy for advanced cancers, before hip replacements and before cataract surgery' because 'the pain and disadvantages caused by not being able to have children is greater than that of most other diseases' (Lilford 1993).

Some infertility specialists have argued that married couples with infertility problems may well have a moral right to use reproductive technologies. The Ethics Committee of the American Fertility Society (of fertility specialists) for example, has claimed that couples have a right to reproduce, including if necessary the right to reproduce with medical assistance. The Committee concluded, 'The married couple's right to reproduce should extend to non-coital means of conception which include the wide range of choices made possible by developments in IVF' (Ethics Committee of the American Fertility Society 1986: 4S).

The dominant public perception which specialists have created of the development of new forms of treatment being primarily a response to desperate demand is reinforced by statements made by infertile women who are indeed desperate for help. One woman has argued, for example, that she would still have undergone IVF even if she had known at the time that the private clinic she attended had not yet had any successful births: 'At least it was a chance and if I didn't do it I would never know whether I had that chance or not' (Lasker and Borg 1989: 57). Other infertile women have talked movingly of the pain of not being able to conceive and give birth to a child of their own. As one infertile woman has explained

> Sometimes I feel very negative about myself. It's not as bad as it used to be, but one of the worst times for me was when I felt terrible about myself as a woman. I felt that I wasn't complete. This was not because I hadn't given birth to a baby, but because something was wrong with me ... that I couldn't have a baby.
>
> (Lewis, in Klein 1989: 23)

Not only are the new reproductive technologies promoted as meeting the needs of individuals or rather married couples suffering from infertility, they are also 'sold' as being of benefit to society as a whole. For example, Robert Edwards and colleagues, arguing in support of their claim for more public spending on infertility treatment programmes, claimed 'It is impossible to put a price on the benefits to society of producing wanted children raised in a caring environment' (1989: 1328).

Infertility experts also hold out the promise of a world free from the horrors of genetically inherited diseases and handicaps. IVF combined with egg donation and embryo transfer is, for example, promoted as the solution to genetically inherited defects. According to Carl Wood

> It may be possible for the test-tube procedure to reduce the incidence of, or eliminate, certain defects from the population. For example, where both partners are carriers of recessive genes that in combination would result in a major birth defect, it may be possible to select eggs and sperm cells that would avoid such a situation.
>
> (Wood, cited by Corea 1988: 128)

Sex selection of embryos within an IVF treatment programme has already been successfully used in Britain to enable a couple to avoid the risk of giving birth to a genetically handicapped boy. One proponent of using sex selection within IVF programmes has even gone beyond arguing that such a technique has 'obvious advantages for couples at risk for X-linked diseases' to suggest that sex selection could in future be used to 'assign birth order' within the family which would, in her opinion, be the 'ultimate family planning' (Carson 1988: 18). It is now quite clear that techniques such as IVF which were originally hailed as the treatment of last resort for the relatively small number of women with severely blocked or damaged fallopian tubes are now being used on a much wider scale. In 1980 one specialist was already arguing 'The biggest population (for external fertilization) are going to be men with low sperm count' (Jacobson, cited by Corea 1988: 121). By the early 1990s the use of IVF and GIFT to help couples whose infertility is primarily due to the man's low sperm count was growing rapidly. Couples with 'unexplained infertility' were also being offered IVF in many clinics (see Hull et al. 1992).

Throughout the 1980s most supporters of IVF/GIFT programmes had to admit – at least within their own specialist journals – that their success rate in terms of creating live healthy babies was rather low. However, by the early 1990s specialists were claiming that their success rates were rising rapidly and one British clinic even claimed in 1992 that if women under 40 with fertility problems persisted with IVF for six or more cycles their prognosis for a live birth 'is at least as good as for fertile couples if they persist with treatment' (Hull *et al.* 1992)

Reproductive technology: an evaluation

The claim made above that reproductive technologies such as IVF are now becoming so successful that they rival the success rate of natural conception is at first sight a major triumph of medical technology and a counterblast to those critics who insist that reproductive technologies are 'failed' technologies. It is certainly true that the success rates of techniques such as IVF have steadily increased as experts become more familiar with them. Nevertheless, the *majority* of infertile couples who undergo techniques such as IVF and GIFT still fail to produce a healthy child of their own. By the end of the 1980s the overall success rate measured in maternities for all well-established IVF clinics in the UK was only 9.7 per cent per couple treated. In other words over 90 per cent of couples given IVF failed to take home a baby at the end of their treatment (Page 1989). Critics of IVF have also expressed concern over the high rates of multiple births it produces. Women having IVF in the 1980s were 27 times more likely to have a multiple birth than the general population (Oakley 1993). By the early 1990s the highest success rates claimed by the larger, more established British clinics in a population of 'carefully selected' couples were only approaching 50 per cent after three cycles of treatment (the point at which most couples are advised to give up). Many smaller clinics still have far lower success rates. It is also significant to note that infertility clinics now offer IVF to couples with unexplained infertility who appear to have 'normal menstrual and ovulation cycles, normal sperm–cervical mucus interaction and normal laparoscopic findings' (Hull *et al.* 1992: 1465). Given that research has demonstrated that 7 to 28 per cent of women accepted for IVF treatment conceive naturally either before starting treatment or within two years of discontinuation (Wagner and St Clair 1989), we need far more randomized controlled clinical trials of the new reproductive technologies before specialists can claim that their treatments are significantly more effective than allowing nature to take its course. Yet doctors themselves have openly admitted, within the relative privacy of their own medical journals, that very few such trials have been carried out on the new reproductive technologies (e.g. Tulandi and Cherry 1989).

The relatively low success rates of technologies such as IVF or GIFT might be completely acceptable to infertile women if the treatments concerned were simple, painless and risk-free. Unfortunately, this is far from being the case. The popular press talk about 'test-tube babies' and IVF is sometimes described as a technique which simply assists nature by mixing a woman's eggs with a man's sperm in a glass dish before putting the embryos back into the woman's body where they/it continue to grow naturally. What is often missed out in this simplified account of IVF is the preparation of the woman's body before her eggs are 'harvested' and the pain and discomfort women usually endure during a series of invasive procedures leading up to the implantation of the embryo in her womb.

Most IVF specialists give women hormonal injections to stimulate her ovaries and control her ovulatory cycles. These injections are time consuming and often painful. Moreover, the drugs used to stimulate ovulation have a wide range of potentially very unpleasant side effects. For example, one woman who was prescribed progressively higher doses of Clomid – one of the drugs routinely prescribed to IVF and GIFT patients in a cocktail with other drugs – has described its relatively common side effects thus:

> I had dizzy spells, a constant pain in the left side of my belly and a funny feeling inside my head . . . I couldn't see sharply any more. I saw lights and colours and I felt kind of strange/funny inside my head.
>
> (Esser, in Klein 1989: 61)

Another unpleasant and often painful part of IVF/GIFT treatment is egg collection. In order to overcome the dangers of using a general anaesthetic to carry out this procedure via a laparoscopy, specialists have developed a new procedure using ultrasound which involves inserting a needle through a woman's full bladder and then into her ovary. Women must lie absolutely still during this procedure which takes at least half an hour. Some experts have admitted that one of the problems with this newer procedure is the pain it causes the patient. An American specialist, for example, has commented that unlike Danish and British women, American women would not accept this procedure because it was too painful. The procedure can also induce heavy bleeding and/or infections but as it is an out-patient procedure it 'lowers the costs of IVF . . . and also accelerates its acceptance as a reimbursable service through health insurance' (Shulman, in Rowland 1992: 28).

Some infertile women may decide that the risk of pain and even a physical illness is still a price worth paying for a baby of their own but sadly there have now been a number of deaths worldwide as a direct result of infertility treatment. There have been reports of deaths of women on IVF programmes in Spain, Brazil, Israel and Australia (Rowland 1992), and in 1993 the first British woman died from the complications of ovarian hyperstimulation syndrome caused by IVF treatment. Her consultant gynaecologist told an inquest that he had not warned her there was any risk of death (*The Guardian*, 25 February 1994). Statistically, such deaths may be totally insignificant but they do highlight the physical risks women face when undergoing fertility treatments which often involve long term drug use and repeated operations. The medical literature pays little attention either to these risks or unpleasant side effects. Women who have undergone IVF treatment, however, tell a different story. One woman, describing her own experience, has written

> Here she is thirty years old, lying with her head down, waiting for the embryo to take, to stick onto the walls of her uterus, to stay . . . Here she is all agony and anguish, all bitterness and heartache, all pain and grief. Here she is debased and degraded, embarrassed and humbled, shamed and subdued. Their guinea pig, their hatching hen, their hormone cow, their willing victim.
>
> (Goldman, in Klein 1989: 70)

As well as the physical traumas imposed by treatments such as IVF, it is also now well-documented that undergoing long term infertility treatment places women, and indeed their partners, under very heavy emotional strain. Some fertility specialists have admitted that IVF treatment imposes great strain on those undergoing it. Robert Winston, for example, has argued that IVF is 'so very fraught emotionally' that many women simply cannot tolerate repeated attempts (Winston and Margara 1987: 785).

One of the many reasons why IVF treatment is so emotionally fraught is that once embarked upon, many women find it very difficult to stop. One woman, when asked whether she had ever considered dropping out of an IVF programme, replied 'It's not a question of choice. You cannot say no to IVF – I think that I would blame myself for the rest of my life if I said no to this last cycle because it might result in a child' (Koch, in Klein 1989: 109). One American specialist has advised other doctors treating infertile couples:

> Our culture worships success and denigrates the quitter. The couple who have not achieved a pregnancy must feel they have exhausted every avenue, have given it their best shot. The term 'give up' must never be used.
>
> (Taylor 1990: 773)

Barbara Rothman has described the inability to give up as 'the burden of not trying hard enough' and has suggested that 'taking away the sense of inevitability' in relation to infertility and 'substituting the "choice" of giving up' does not in any real sense increase such couples' choice and control (Rothman 1984: 31).

Feminist critics of reproductive technologies have also pointed out that they reinforce the cult of motherhood in male-dominated societies. For example, according to one leading infertility specialist, 'It is a fact that there is a biological drive to reproduce. Women who deny this drive or in whom it is frustrated show disturbances in other ways' (Steptoe, cited by Stanworth 1987: 15) Gena Corea has argued that this dominant view of infertile women as not proper women, which many infertile women themselves feel very strongly,

> has a coercive power. It conditions a woman's choices as well as the motivation to choose. Her most heartfelt desire, the pregnancy for which she so desperately yearns has been – to varying degrees – conditioned.

This conditioning tells women from a very early age that 'We are here to bear the children of men. If we cannot do it we are not real women. There is no reason for us to exist' (Corea 1988: 17).

Infertility specialists emphasize in public that they are simply responding to the needs of those suffering from a very painful illness. However, many of those providing high-tech forms of infertility treatment are not just doctors but research scientists. Their work is designed to take them to the very edge of medical scientific knowledge, and beyond. A number of leading specialists have openly written of their excitement in being involved in this quest for new knowledge. One doctor working on egg donation and its application in reproductive technologies has written, for example, 'the great challenge and possible reward of a donor oocyte program will be the scientific information derived from these clinical experiments' (Rosenwaks 1987: 895). According to Patricia Spallone, scientists may argue in public that IVF is all about meeting women's needs but their thinking is actually 'centred on themselves' and 'what it means for science'. In support of this claim Spallone cited Edwards, describing his first 'successful pregnancy' using IVF which was actually an ectopic pregnancy:

> At long last in 1975 the first successful pregnancy was established . . . What a wonderful moment! But it ended in disappointment, because it was an ectopic pregnancy, implanted in the oviduct and the fetus died and had to be removed. But this was a wonderful stimulus to us, even though the pregnancy ended tragically. We knew that our embryos were capable of implanting. . .
>
> (Edwards, cited by Spallone 1989: 101)

Lasker and Borg who interviewed a number of infertility specialists observed that, whilst they often worked very hard to help infertile couples, many of them were also 'ambitious go-getters' who were primarily motivated by 'the challenge of working at the frontiers of science and by the prestige of being at the top of their field'. One director of a fertility clinic told them, 'Personally, it is important to me that the work I do helps women. But by far the most exciting part professionally is the research and the new data we get' (Lasker and Borg 1989: 130).

Women are pulled into medical research programmes with the carrot of the possibility of pregnancy followed by a live birth but in the very recent past many women have been misled as to the likelihood that they themselves would take home a live healthy baby. Ironically Lesley Brown, much fêted as the mother of the world's first 'test-tube' baby, has explained how she did not at first realize that no woman before her had ever produced a baby via IVF. She has described her first meeting with Patrick Steptoe thus:

> I don't remember Mr Steptoe saying his method of producing babies had ever worked and I certainly didn't ask. I just imagined that hundreds of children had already been born through being conceived outside their mother's womb.
>
> (Corea 1988: 167)

Other women who have undergone experimental treatment for infertility have also testified that they had very unrealistic expectations of its likely outcome. One young Danish woman, for example, joined an experimental IVF programme believing that it would give her a better chance of becoming pregnant than if she joined a 'regular' IVF programme. She was therefore extremely shocked to learn from a technician after she had undergone three cycles of treatment that no one had ever become pregnant from the treatment given to the women in her experimental group (Klein 1989: 105).

Using infertile women as part of scientific experiments surely raises ethical issues, particularly if their informed consent is not obtained. Yet, as Patricia Spallone has pointed out, the ethical debate surrounding the new reproductive technologies has focused primarily on the use of embryos rather than the use of women's bodies. According to Spallone

> Ignoring women and talking in terms of embryos is morally less problematic than admitting that women are the subject of 'human IVF' and 'human embryo' experimentation. It is much easier to deal with the ethics of experimentation with embryos rather than the ethics of experimenting with women's bodies.
>
> (1989: 22)

Some infertile women have argued that they are quite prepared to join scientific experiments in return for even a slim chance of becoming pregnant. Barbara Menning made the following plea to the fertile in 1981:

> Let those of us who are infertile decide whether we are willing to subject ourselves to the instrumentation and intervention necessary to unite ovum and sperm and reimplant the conceptus in our bodies. Let us make informed consent, since we will incur the risks.
>
> (Menning 1981: 264)

At first reading this is a very persuasive argument. The problem, however, lies with the notion of informed consent. Even some fertility specialists themselves now openly admit that some of their colleagues have misled potential patients. For example, in 1987 a group of American specialists admitted

> Infertile patients often develop unrealistically high expectations regarding specific therapies. The medical community is partly responsible for these inflated expectations when practitioners claim pregnancy rates that far exceed those found in the current literature.
>
> (Blackwell *et al.* 1987: 737)

It is not just women with fertility problems who may be misled by medical researchers. Rowland suggests that some women who were asked to donate their eggs in order to 'help infertile couples have children' may well have donated eggs which researchers used for embryo experimentation without the donors' informed consent (Rowland 1992).

The drive for new knowledge and the prestige which comes from being first in a medical research race are by no means the only factors behind the rapid development and expansion of high technology infertility treatments. These new treatments are also highly profitable and are seen by many businesspeople to have the potential to become very big business indeed. This aspect of the new reproductive technologies may be somewhat hidden in Britain where public concern has been primarily focused on the ethics of these new treatments and the very limited free access to them currently provided by the NHS. By 1993 there were only six fully funded NHS infertility units in Britain and long queues had formed for free IVF treatment (Lilford 1993). Some health authorities were attempting to remove IVF from the list of medical treatments they were prepared to fund for their local population (Redmayne and Klein 1993). Understandably such patchy public provision caused great distress to those infertile couples who were unable to afford the £1,500 average cost of one cycle of IVF treatment in the private sector. Worldwide, however, debates over IVF and other new forms of infertility treatment have included serious concern over the extent to which infertile couples may be being exploited by this new growth industry. Whilst medical treatment is not inevitably exploitative simply because it is being provided on a for-profit basis, even infertility specialists themselves have recognized that infertile couples may be particularly vulnerable to exploitation by private infertility clinics. In 1987 an article in *Fertility and Sterility* entitled 'Are we exploiting the infertile couple?' listed three key ways in which such exploitation could occur. First, they claimed that in the United States it was becoming commonplace

> for practitioners to visit academic or private IVF programs for a short time and then return to their hospitals and attempt to open IVF or GIFT programs. The motive for establishing such programs may not be a strong interest in IVF or the desire to fill a void in the community but an attempt by a hospital corporation to increase its market share.
>
> (Blackwell *et al.* 1987: 737)

Second, the authors suggested, IVF was sometimes being used before a complete evaluation of the couple's infertility problem had been carried out and that too often in a consumer-driven, for-profit health care system doctors offered 'premature or indiscriminate therapy' to those who demanded it, rather than risk losing the patient to 'a more accommodating competitor'. Finally, the authors expressed concern over claims by some specialists that they had achieved pregnancy rates far in excess of those found in the current medical literature. They argued that 'to quote a high pregnancy rate based on young patients with only tubal disease and apply it to patients of all ages and diagnoses is deceptive' (Blackwell *et al.* 1987: 738).

In 1989 an editorial in *Fertility and Sterility* entitled 'Truth in advertising' noted that in the US in 1988 'less than one-half of IVF programs had yet to produce a live birth' (Younger 1989: 726). Yet private clinics there were free to advertise their IVF programs in highly emotive and completely inexplicit terms. The editorial then cited the following advertisement

> There is no other perfume like it, the smell of a newborn: a milk scent, warm-scent, cuddle essence. Her skin a kind of new velvet. Toes more wrinkled than cabbage, yet roselike. Tender, soft, totally trusting: a blessing all of your own. That dream might still come true for you. New techniques can resolve many infertility problems, including some that were previously considered hopeless. Before you let go of the dream, talk to us.
>
> (Younger 1989: 727)

The commercialization of infertility treatment has reached almost bizarre extremes in some countries. One Australian IVF clinic, for example, has offered IVF treatment to Asians as part of a holiday package. Its director has argued, 'What could be more natural than to go for a month's holiday and when you come back, be pregnant' (Rowland 1992: 221). In Britain private infertility clinics may be less inventive in their search for paying patients but one leading infertility specialist who does no private work himself has expressed serious concern over the service some of these clinics provide. According to Professor Robert Winston the standard of infertility treatment in Britain is generally not good and in the private sector 'there is a huge amount of shocking practice' (Winston cited by Levin 1991).

IVF treatment has not only proved highly profitable for doctors offering it within the private health care sector, it has also proved a boon for drugs and medical equipment manufacturers. In 1982 the sales of the drug Perganol – used in infertility treatment – were $7.2 million; by 1986 they had risen to $35 million. Meanwhile, one American company, which was given a patent on instruments to harvest fertilized human eggs estimated that IVF could become 'a $6 billion annual business' but only – as a reporter from *The New York Times* pointed out – if IVF clinics learnt to made a lot more babies (Rowland 1992: 218).

Whilst the drive for profits may be most clear cut within the private health care sector, even infertility specialists and researchers working within the public sector usually have a close relationship – directly or indirectly – with the private companies which supply the equipment and drugs needed to turn scientists' dreams into reality. The chairman of the American Fertility Society's Industry Committee urged his medical colleagues in 1988 not to ignore 'the substantial sustaining' support they received from the industry:

> Aside from the financial support, we receive a more vital support from industry for the success of our individual professional practices. The corporations that support the American Fertility Society translate our needs for patient care into products that meet those needs. Without this corporate support there would be no laparoscopy, no sonography, no laser therapy, no in vitro fertilization.
>
> (Bates 1988: 398)

One is tempted to complete the other half of this equation thus: 'Without laparoscopy etc. there would be no large corporate profits.'

The Professor of Obstetrics and Gynaecology who directed the original research into the use of donor eggs within an IVF programme has claimed that without private financing such research would not be possible. He has also admitted that Wall Street demands a good return on its investment:

> Wall Street will never help you unless they get their money out ... You have to understand that getting money out of it is what makes their system work for them, even though that relationship compromises some of the dear academic principles we've always espoused.
>
> (Buster in Lasker and Borg 1989: 105)

Whilst high technology treatments for infertility have proved highly profitable and have found ample backing from private industry, research into the causes of infertility is far less well funded. Infertility specialists now tend to refer to infertility as a 'terrible disease' and argue that those suffering from it have a right to treatment. However, these pioneers of IVF and GIFT rarely refer to the need to investigate why women – and men – come to be suffering from this disease in the first place. For example, pelvic inflammatory disease (PID) is a major cause of tubal damage in women, yet very little priority is given within the health services to the prevention and treatment of this common problem (Mosse and Heaton 1990: 215) The prevention and treatment of sexually transmitted diseases which can cause PID is simply not a prestigious high status medical speciality. Whereas Patrick Steptoe became a famous public figure after 'producing' the first test-tube babies, specialists in venereal diseases are hardly likely to become public heroes.

Whilst the medical profession and health services might do more to prevent infertility, some causes of infertility lie outside the remit of modern medicine. There is evidence, for example, that certain chemicals, found predominantly in the workplace can adversely affect male and female fertility (see Spallone 1989: 74). Severe poverty too can lead to women being unable to bear and raise healthy children. Yet far from demanding more support for poor parents some infertility specialists have even argued that one of the advantages of assisted reproduction is that it can ensure that only adults who can afford to support them are given the chance to have babies (see Wood, in Klein 1989).

Critics of the new reproductive technologies are not solely concerned with their current impact on women and their potential for exploiting the infertile. A number of feminist writers have written of their fears that the ever-increasing use of these technologies will continue to suck more and more women into a highly medicalized and controlling form of conception, pregnancy and childbirth. Already, infertility specialists have rapidly expanded the types of infertility problems deemed to be curable by IVF/GIFT. Women who have no infertility problems of their own are now being subjected to IVF in order to give their subfertile male partners the chance of a child who genetically belongs to them. A significant number of women seeking IVF treatment are not even childless. They have already borne children but then change partners and cannot naturally give their new partner a child of his own. One women who had three children from a previous marriage explained why she was undergoing IVF thus: 'My husband John doesn't have any children of his own . . . I'm doing this for him' (Corea, 1985: 171).

Women whose male partners suffer from infertility could become pregnant using the much simpler and less invasive technique of artificial insemination by donor (AID) but their male partners may not find such a solution acceptable. Couples with fertility problems interviewed by Judith Lasker and Susan Borg who had rejected adoption both cited the desire for a biological child as the reason. But according to Lasker and Borg, 'men usually appear to be the driving force behind the preference for a biological child. Many women told us they would by happy to adopt but that their husbands wanted a genetic connection' (1989: 16).

Whilst society, and indeed fertile women, themselves, seem to accept as natural men's drive to produce a biological child of their own, society appears far less happy to accept the idea that women who do not have a heterosexual relationship may also have a drive to become mothers. Since the early 1980s a few women have bypassed medicalized forms of assisted reproduction and turned to a do-it-yourself method of becoming pregnant – artificial insemination by donor. In 1980, for example, six women in London organized themselves into 'The Feminist Self-Insemination Group'. By 1983 they had sold more than 1,000 copies of their pamphlet which explained the self-insemination process and British women had conceived several children through self-insemination (Klein 1984). In the US a number of feminist health care clinics have offered a donor insemination service since the late 1970s. Such clinics have been adamant that the process should be as demedicalized as possible and that doctors should play no part in deciding whether a woman is 'suitable' for donor insemination. These services have allowed disabled women, single women, lesbian women and women of colour equal access to a fertility service otherwise controlled and rationed by the medical profession (see Hornstein 1984).

Perhaps not surprisingly, legislators and the medical profession have been extremely unhappy about the existence of do-it-yourself assisted insemination. The Warnock Committee, for example, recommended that any non-licensed donor insemination should be a criminal activity (Warnock 1985). In the US it is already a criminal offence in several states to perform AID without a medical licence. Why have women's attempts to use a very simple method of assisted conception without having to submit to medical control and supervision caused such outrage? Why, for example, did the British press launch a moral panic in 1991 over the use of donor insemination by a 'virgin' or rather by a woman who had not had sex with a man? According to *The Daily Mail* (11 March 1991), donor insemination by women who do not have sex by men 'strikes at the very heart of family life'. MP Ann Winterton described the practice as 'immoral and unnatural'. Stephen Green on the Conservative Family Campaign said it was 'repellent and selfish'. According to feminists, the real threat to society of self-insemination is that it strikes at the very heart of male control over women. As one fearful journalist put it 'Are men now redundant?'

Whilst some women who do not themselves suffer from the 'disease' of infertility have been pulled into IVF programmes to meet the desires of their male partners, other women who have been desperate to have a child of their own have been deemed unsuitable for motherhood by the medical gatekeepers to IVF programmes. Although neither the British nor the American medical profession has ruled out helping single women to conceive, virtually all IVF specialists have restricted their services to heterosexual couples in long term stable relationships. In 1983 the Ethics Committee of the Royal College of Obstetricians and Gynaecologists stated in their guidelines on IVF, that doctors could refuse access to treatment on social as well as medical grounds (RCOG 1983). The Committee advised that IVF should only be used for single women in 'exceptional circumstances'. In 1987 a patient's guide to infertility treatment published by the British Medical Association (BMA) asked, can a single woman ask for IVF? It replied,

> She can ask but most units will refuse her. Many feminist groups feel that it is a woman's right to have a child when she wants and in the way she wants, but society and clinicians find it difficult to offer such an expensive, complex, and extremely demanding treatment to single women while 12% or more of stable couples are trying so hard to have children to bring up within the family.
>
> (Leila and Elliot 1987: 10)

Many AID clinics, particularly publicly funded clinics, also restrict access to heterosexual couples only and even then such couples may have to undergo several interviews to assess their stability and emotional maturity before being accepted for help. Lesbian women wanting to conceive a child through AID have either used a do-it-yourself method, thus avoiding the control of the medical profession altogether, or they have turned to the very few clinics which are non-discriminatory.

Although there is as yet very little published research on how assessment of eligibility for IVF treatment is carried out in practice, it is clear that at least within the public sector in Britain, couples must fulfil a range of social as well as medical criteria. For example, in order to get onto the waiting list for treatment at one NHS clinic offering IVF, a woman must be less than 36, a man less than 46. The couple must have lived together for at least three years and must fulfil adoption criteria. One woman was removed from the waiting list for IVF on the NHS because she had a conviction for offences related to prostitution and had previously been rejected as a potential foster or adoptive parent by the local social services department. This woman attempted to use the courts to challenge this decision but the judge ruled that the unit's decision was neither unfair nor unreasonable (Douglas *et al.* 1992).

Not only are medical experts already deciding which infertile women fit the social criteria deemed appropriate for 'their' mothers, they are also actively searching for other types of women to act as surrogates and egg donors within their reproductive programmes. One proponent of egg donation has concluded that the largest source of eggs will have to be 'women recruited specifically for egg donation' and argued that he could see no ethical objections to paying poorer women to become egg donors. He went on to dismiss the feminist argument that poor women were likely to be exploited as egg donors on two grounds. First, the recipients' desire to receive good genes would 'place a premium on women who are healthy and appear to be of good stock'. Second, neither the risks nor payments would be so great 'that an unacceptable exploitation of poorer persons would occur' (Robertson 1989: 360). In Britain a private London clinic advertised for egg donors in the early 1990s with advertisements for women under 35 to become anonymous egg donors in order to provide 'the ultimate gift – the gift of life'. Despite the gruelling regime involved in donating eggs the clinic did not offer any payment to its volunteers (*The Observer*, 19 January 1992). Another private British clinic encouraged young childless women to donate eggs in return for free infertility treatment but one specialist condemned the idea saying 'This concept smacks of bringing undue pressure on people to give away their own eggs in exchange for free treatment when they need the eggs themselves' (Brinsden cited by Rogers 1993).

As well as pulling women into assisted reproduction programmes as egg donors some infertility specialists are also keen to explore all forms of surrogacy. One Australian specialist in reproductive physiology is even reported as saying that a woman who was brain-dead could be used as a surrogate mother or surrogate womb. He reportedly claimed, 'it is a wonderful solution to the problems posed by surrogacy and a magnificent use of a corpse. It has my complete support' (Gerber, cited by Rowland 1992: 198). The surrogacy industry has already paid poor women to have babies for rich couples. Once specialists improve the technique of embryo transfer more women will be used to bear the fertilized eggs of other women and the potential of the surrogate industry will be much greater. One American baby broker has predicted that eventually the industry will use surrogates from the Third World in order to lower the costs of the service. He was even thinking of just paying such surrogates travel and living expenses rather than a fee on the grounds that 'often they're looking for a survival situation – something to do to pay for the rent and food (Stethura, cited by Corea 1985: 245).

Most discussions of the potential impact of the new reproductive technologies, including feminist analyses, have limited their explorations to affluent capitalist countries. Renate Klein, however, has expressed strong fears about the impact of these technologies on women in Third World countries. She fears, for example, that IVF programmes could be linked to population control programmes and cites two Indian IVF specialists who claimed that test-tube baby technology could have a 'promotive effect' on the country's family planning programme as it showed the successful reversal of sterilization techniques. Klein comments, 'We can be sure however that in the same way as in the West only "respectable" women gain access to IVF, sterilization reversal for the poor landless peasant women will not become a priority' (1989: 271).

It is certainly becoming clearer – as the use of reproductive technologies expands rapidly – that the costs of such treatments will mean that only a minority of women with fertility problems worldwide will ever gain access to them. Women thus face a double jeopardy. Poor women and women from ethnic minority groups may be denied the medical help they need to conceive a baby of their own whilst being pulled into reproductive technology pro-grammes as egg donors or surrogate baby carriers. White affluent married women on the other hand may also be pulled into assisted reproduction programmes as recipients of medical assistance even though they would be perfectly able to conceive a child of their own without any such 'help'. Research scientists are now beginning to hold out the possibility of using reproductive technologies to prevent genetically transmitted diseases and defects. Renate Klein fears that the range of 'disabilities' to be 'cured' in this way could expand indefinitely and might eventually include traits simply considered undesirable by society, such as homosexuality (Klein 1989: 265). Equally alarming is the prospect in the not too distant future of any woman who wishes to conceive a baby the natural non-medicalized way being told by her doctor that her selfishness might put her child at risk of a whole range of genetic defects. Virtually all women could – under such circumstances – have their reproductive lives more or less totally controlled by the medical profession. In 1985 Gena Corea looked into the future and painted a picture of a reproductive brothel in which most women would be defined as 'non-valuable' and sterilized and in this way their progeny culled . . . In the United States women of colour would probably be labelled 'non-valuable' and used as breeders for the embryos of valuable women. White women judged genetically superior would be selected as egg donors and thus turned into machines for producing embryos.

(Corea 1985: 45)

Such a horrifying prediction might be dismissed as loony feminist science fiction if it were not for the fact that many elements of Corea's 'fantasy' can be found in the statements and actions of those who currently control the new reproductive technologies. According to Professor Carl Wood, for example,

Natural conception compares less favourably than artificial conception as it includes unwanted children, parents incapable of parenting, poverty-stricken parents and women with medical diseases or habits likely to adversely affect the child.

(Klein 1989: 267)

In 1971 the retiring President of the American Association for the Advancement of Science argued that eventually every child should have a right 'to be born with a sound physical and mental constitution based on a sound genotype. No parents will in that future time have a right to burden society with a malformed or a mentally incompetent child' (cited in Scutt 1988: 218).

Conclusion

It is not easy to resist demands for more public funding for high technology infertility treatments when specialists make emotive appeals on behalf of desperate childless couples who, they claim, are suffering from a terrible but curable disease. It is even harder to resist appeals from women themselves who have talked of their despair and resentment at seeing those with enough money jumping the queue for IVF treatment. One woman waiting for NHS treatment has said

If I could pay I might well have a baby by now . . . I don't think people realize how upsetting it is especially when you see foreign and other women signing cheques and jumping in ahead of you. I can't blame the hospital but I feel somehow I am being punished.

(Doyle 1991)

A major increase in NHS funding for high technology infertility units might at least ensure women more equal access to the chance of conceiving a baby. Lesley Doyal has argued, for example,

Unless expenditure on the NHS is increased, the current trend towards commercialisation will continue and many women will be forced to go without or to go outside the service for treatment. As a result the gap between the rich and poor will continue to widen, and the chance of a baby will become a 'commodity' available only to the prosperous infertile.

(1987: 187)

However, even if the new reproductive technologies were to become far more successful in delivering live, healthy babies than their current rather low success rate, and even if purchasers within the NHS decided that such treatments did offer relatively good value for money, they would still be extremely costly in terms of women's own physical and emotional well-being. One ardent critic of these new technologies has suggested

When accused of being callous towards women who desperately desire to have children, we must respond by raising the spectre of the real inhumanity that reproductive technologies force upon women. It is not callous or inhumane to ask why women are channelled, at such a cost to themselves, into reproducing.

(Raymond 1984: 435)

Infertile women could well respond to this argument by insisting that they should be allowed to choose for themselves whether to undergo physically and emotionally draining treatment in the hope of becoming biological mothers, but this option will never be open to those women with fertility problems who are deemed by those who control these technologies to be unsuitable for parenthood. Unsuitability can be based on a woman's age, her sexual preference, her sexual history and above all her income – or rather her lack of it. Whereas male film stars in their 60s and 70s are hailed as virility symbols when they father a child, post-menopausal women in their early 50s are labelled as supremely selfish when they achieve the same feat with a donor egg. Despite society's disapproval, very rich older women can usually purchase what they want – even a baby of their own. The majority of very poor infertile women in both western capitalist countries and developing countries will never be able to afford the chance to be 'helped' by reproductive technologies. Perhaps the most disturbing aspect of these new technologies, however, is neither the false promises and heavy burdens they impose on those who use them nor the issue of unequal access to them, but their growing impact over the whole process of conception, pregnancy and childbirth and therefore on the concept of motherhood itself. On balance, the dangers potentially posed to all women by the ever-expanding, highly profitable programmes of assisted reproduction and genetic engineering may well soon outweigh the undoubted benefits gained by those relatively small numbers of women who finally achieve the baby of their dreams through the use of medical technologies. In any case there are alternative approaches to the very real pain caused by infertility within our society. Simple measures which might reduce the incidence of infertility in developed countries are left unimplemented by an indifferent medical profession and societies in which the pursuit of profits takes precedence over the meeting of human need. Similarly, simple and very cheap self-help measures such as do-it-yourself AID are opposed by many medical experts and condemned as immoral by male dominated societies which seem to be fearful of women controlled forms of infertility treatment. It is this overt hostility to women meeting their own reproductive needs without any medical assistance which highlights so clearly the issue of control over female reproduction. One does not have to believe in male conspiracies nor assume that all fertility specialists are primarily interested in money or prestige to recognize that to date the development of the new reproductive technologies has increased medical control over women's reproductive lives and improved the profits of the health care industry while doing little to help the majority of women suffering from impaired fertility. Nor does one have to be a completely paranoid woman to worry that perhaps Renate Klein was not just wildly scaremongering when she warned in 1985

> Among the things the next 'wave' of the women's movement might have to fight for could be a woman's right to bear her own natural children: we could have lost control over the last part of the reproductive process to decide if, when and how to conceive, carry and give birth to children.

> (1985: 71)

4

THE MENOPAUSE

Sometime towards the end of the twentieth century the menopause came out of the closet and a previously unmentionable topic of polite conversation finally became almost fashionable. Feminists who had earlier written books about sex and childbirth reached that 'certain age' and began to pay attention to the climacteric. Germaine Greer, to take a leading example, moved on from writing about sex in the 1960s and motherhood in the 1980s to produce *The Change: Women, Ageing and the Menopause* (1992) – a new feminist text for the 1990s. Meanwhile, British women in the public eye including the British actress Kate O'Mara and the politician Theresa Gorman actively campaigned for hormone replacement therapy (HRT) to be made far more widely available to British women. In the late 1980s it was even rumoured that Margaret Thatcher was on HRT. The popular press began to publish pro-HRT articles with titles such as 'Everything you need to know about the drug therapy that can help a woman stay young'. Even decidedly pre-menopausal women began to worry about whether or not they would benefit from this new wonder drug. The British medical profession remained – on the whole – somewhat cautious in their prescribing of HRT but a growing number of British medical experts publicly endorsed the view that the menopause was a treatable deficiency disease.

In this chapter the shift in medical and public opinion from conceptualizing the menopause as a relatively uneventful natural occurrence in 'normal' women to defining it as a universal but treatable deficiency disease will be outlined. The claims made by the promoters of HRT will then be critically evaluated and the known side effects and dangers of this type of treatment assessed. Finally, the view that women's menopausal problems are as much a political as a medical issue will be explored. First, however, we will briefly describe what is known about the menopause and its effects.

As a woman ages her ovaries begin to slow down and the levels of oestrogen in her body become more irregular. Less progesterone is produced and eventually, usually after a long period of irregular menstrual cycles, menstruation ceases altogether. Every woman's climacteric is different but the perimenopausal period usually lasts for very approximately 10 years and most frequently occurs between the ages of 45 and 55. Although many medical texts authoritatively list the symptoms which can occur during the climacteric, one has only to read a few such texts to realize that medical experts cannot agree on which of the many problems middle-aged women tend to present to their doctors are directly caused by the menopause and which are rather caused by ageing or life events unconnected to the physiological changes of the climacteric. According to one medical article on the menopause its symptoms include flushes and sweats, dizziness, palpitations, migraine headaches, atrophic vaginitis, urethral syndrome (frequency, urgency dysuria), mood changes, irritability, depression, agoraphobia, panic attacks, loss of confidence, poor concentration, tiredness/fatigue, declining memory and mental faculties, indecisiveness, loss of self esteem, joint pains, stiffness, loss of libido and dyspareunia (Gangar and Key 1991). Reading such a list one is amazed that any menopausal woman can still stand upright let alone hold down a full time job or run a household. Other medical experts, however, strongly dispute the view that psychological problems such as depression or agoraphobia are causally linked to the physiological changes which do occur during the climacteric (see Hunter *et al* 1986). The only two problems which experts appear to agree are conclusively linked to the menopause are hot flushes and vaginal atrophy. Hot flushes are usually explained as being caused by declining levels of oestrogen, but even this simple statement is not conclusive. Indeed, according to Germaine Greer, scientific knowledge of what happens to a woman's hormones during the climacteric is most notable for its absence. Greer points out that even the most clear cut menopausal symptom – flushing – turns out to be a bit of a mystery. In 1976 an article in *The Lancet* revealed that 'no correlation has so far been established between hormonal changes and menopausal flushing . . . we contend there is no clear-cut relation between hot flushes and oestrogen deficiency' (Greer 1992: 176). This may surprise many women and indeed many doctors. Nevertheless Greer's review of experts' knowledge of the menopause concluded that we do not know what is happening, we do not know why it happens, we do not know why some women suffer from some symptoms and others different symptoms, or if it is true that some experience no symptoms at all, we do not know which menopausal symptoms are primarily physical, which psychosomatic and which psychological. According to Greer 'the menopausal muddle is part of the general fog of incomprehension about the health status of middle-aged women' (1992: 183). Yet doctors continue, as they always have done, to give female patients authoritative advice on a subject they actually know remarkably little about but for which, they now increasingly assume, they have a very effective and safe form of treatment.

Menopause: a natural life event

Before HRT became a panacea for menopausal problems, the medical profession adopted the view that 'normal' women should experience few, if any, menopausal symptoms. The menopause was to be viewed as a natural life event rather like puberty but with perhaps more negative connotations. Kimbrough's *Gynecology* (1965: 97) stated, for example, 'All women undergo physiologic changes during the time of the menopause but relatively few are seriously disturbed by them'. Similarly, Jeffcoate's *Principles of Gynaecology* claimed

> In the well adjusted and well informed woman psychological changes are few and insignificant amounting to no more than a period of slight emotional instability followed by the development of the dignity, tolerance, placidity and assurance of old age.
>
> (1957: 93)

Some textbooks even went so far as to emphasize the positive side of the menopause, for example, according to Novak's *Textbook of Gynecology* of 1956

> the cessation of the menstrual function associated as it often is with an increase in weight has converted many an unattractive thin worried woman into the graceful and serene type of matron, veritably a second flowering.
>
> (1956: 632)
>
> (NB: post-Twiggy textbooks are far less sanguine about weight gain during the menopause as indeed are most climacteric women themselves.)

Whilst emphasizing the essentially natural and benign characteristics of the menopause *per se*, 'traditional' medical textbooks nevertheless conveyed a very negative picture of the natural changes most women could expect. For example, Shaw claimed 'the climacteric is thus a phase of adjustment between active and inactive sexual function' (1956: 89). Not only did older women face a loss of sexual desire they also, according to several textbooks, faced the loss of one of their primary roles, if not *the* primary role, in their life, mothering. According to Crossen (1953), for example, a woman's loss of 'mother love' could leave her 'without a substitute'. Loss of sex, loss of motherhood and to cap it all loss of feminine charms, since, during the climacteric; 'the hair becomes grey, the skin loses its subcutaneous fat and develops a sag under the chin and over the face and at the same time fat deposits occur where least desired' (Crossen 1953: 882).

The second key feature of the natural life event medical model of the menopause was that most women going through it, whilst not deemed to need actual medical treatment, were seen as in need of expert medical advice and lifestyle counselling. Doctors and students reading medical texts on the menopause in the 1950s and 60s were strongly encouraged to see themselves as wise, sympathetic advisers to confused, ignorant female patients. Shaw advised in 1956 'it should be emphasized that most menopausal patients need no treatment apart from the tactful handling of a sympathetic doctor and a little help in adjusting themselves' (Shaw 1956: 93). Similarly, Kimbrough claimed in 1965 that in most women 'the flushes and the manifestations of anxiety are mild, often mitigated by sympathetic consultation alone' (Kimbrough 1965: 97).

If paternalistic counselling did not single-handedly dispel all menopausal symptoms, doctors were advised to offer advice on changes to women's lifestyles. Wharton (1943: 197) suggested

> most women notice the hot flushes more when they are tired or worried. Hence, a period of rest every day and freedom from physical and mental fatigue are helpful. Some women are too active in civic and domestic roles, curtailing their overactivities may bring a great deal of relief.

Ten years later, Crossen was suggesting a rather different line of advice;

> the shifting aims of life during this period should be explained, emphasizing that one should not try to deny her age and seek eternal youth by artificial means and alcoholic stimulants but should concentrate her energies on new avenues of service ... Time which is no longer required for family duties can be utilised in other worthwhile family, civic or social projects.
>
> (1953: 883)

The third feature of the natural life event medical model of the menopause was that the small minority of women who experienced more severe medical problems during the climacteric were to be regarded as primarily emotionally unbalanced and/or psychiatrically ill. For example, Shaw advised 'most patients with severe menopausal symptoms are psychically disturbed' (1956: 93) whilst Crossen cited Greenhill's claim that 'psychoneurotic tendencies are apt to be aggravated in the climacteric' (Crossen 1953: 885). 'Highly strung' women were deemed to need sedatives to ease their menopausal symptoms. Wharton claimed

> if a woman is so highly strung and tense that she cannot relax or rest sedation is invaluable. The hot flushes and nervousness will usually decrease as the patient relaxes. The most satisfactory sedatives are bromides and the barbiturates.
>
> (1943: 197)

Some much more recent medical textbooks continue to recommend tranquillizers for some menopausal symptoms. For example, in *Women's Problems in General Practice* Jean Coope (1987) still recommends benzodiazepines in small doses for short periods for 'controlling anxiety and insomnia' during the climacteric.

Whilst no one could accuse this older medical model of the menopause as over-medicalizing most women's lives, it clearly contained a number of negative features when viewed from the patients' perspective. First, much of the information and advice given to menopausal women by their doctors was wrong. For example, it is now generally accepted that there is absolutely no scientific evidence to support the claim that the majority of menopausal and post-menopausal women lose their libido (see Kaplan 1974: 111). Second, the pseudo-medical advice given to women about how to lead the latter part of their lives was clearly at best patronizing and at worst overtly controlling. Third, women suffering severe menopausal symptoms were likely to be stigmatized as innately neurotic if not absolutely mad. Finally, the traditional medical experts, whilst themselves knowing very little of real value about the menopause, totally denied the validity of women's own knowledge and experiences. For example, Shaw's *Textbook of Gynaecology* (1956: 93) stated

> like dysmenorrhoea the menopause is largely bedeviled with old wives' tales and the patient is psychologically conditioned into a state of anxiety neurosis by the case histories, told with painstaking detail, of her friends and relations.

It does seem ironic that whilst women's own wealth of experience of living through the menopause was rudely dismissed as 'old wives' tales' student doctors were encouraged to see themselves as experts on the matter after reading just a chapter or two on the menopause in an ill-informed medical textbook.

Women who consulted doctors who took – and in many cases still take – this 'natural life event' approach to the menopause tended to be caught between the devil and the deep blue sea. Either their extremely debilitating physical symptoms were brushed aside with an 'it's your age, you will have to learn to live with it' or their symptoms were interpreted as psychosomatic, in which case they were treated as neurotic. It is hardly surprising therefore that when Wendy Cooper first published *No Change* in 1975 advocating HRT, older women wrote to her in their thousands complaining bitterly of the ways in which their doctors had responded to their menopausal symptoms. One woman wrote

> I am forty eight and have started the menopause and I get so depressed. I've been to my doctor over hot flushes and sweating and sleeplessness at night, but he doesn't take much notice, just says it's natural and gives me tranquillizers to keep me quiet.
>
> (Cooper 1979: 140)

Given such frustration and even despair it is understandable that so many older women were delighted when a number of British gynaecologists and GPs began to adopt a new approach to the menopause, an approach which regarded it primarily as a deficiency disease which could be very successfully treated with hormone replacement therapy (HRT).

Menopause as a deficiency disease

Hormone replacement therapy is a surprisingly long standing treatment of severe menopausal symptoms. Medical textbooks written in the 1940s advocated the use of hormone treatment for hot flushes and other severe menopausal symptoms if, but only if, all other forms of treatment failed. It was not until the late 1960s that some American doctors began to advocate much more widespread use of HRT. In 1966 Dr Robert Wilson, an American gynaecologist, funded by the drugs industry, hit the bestseller list with his book *Feminine Forever* in which he fervently argued the case for treating the menopause as a 'preventable and curable deficiency disease'. His claim that virtually all menopausal symptoms were physically caused, and were certainly not psychosomatic, was a great comfort to all those older women who had been labelled as mad or neurotic by unsympathetic doctors trained to see extreme menopausal symptoms as a sign of mental rather than physical instability. Moreover, Wilson's belief that HRT could not only cure specific menopausal symptoms but could also delay and diminish visible signs of ageing such as thinning hair and wrinkled skin and thus keep older women looking 'feminine forever' understandably had a strong appeal to women facing up to growing older in an ageist/sexist society.

The claim that the menopause and its symptoms were primarily a deficiency disease was soon adopted enthusiastically by a significant body of American medical opinion. Throughout the 1970s and 1980s, however, the majority of the British medical profession still appeared sceptical of HRT and reluctant to accept the deficiency disease approach to the menopause as the basis for the treatment of all menopausal patients. Nevertheless, this approach did gain gradual acceptance within the UK. In 1979, for example, Wendy Cooper cited the views of a Welsh consultant, Dr Mansel Aylward, who wrote

> simply stated, I consider the climacteric, the menopausal period and the post-menopausal period to be manifestations of a deficiency disease. I use the term disease specifically to indicate that I do not consider it normal that women should be allowed to continue a life with the absence of a substance which is essential for their normal physiology. My analogy, one would not consider preventing patients with diabetes or melitis or Addison's disease receiving the respective hormone replacement therapy, and why should we consider the menopause as anything less than a hormone deficiency disease.
>
> (Cooper 1979: 159)

Whilst few British doctors have accepted the view that virtually all menopausal women should be prescribed HRT, many more GPs are now prepared to consider recommending HRT to at least some of their older female patients. Jean Coope in *Women's Problems in General Practice* typifies the new British approach. She advises GPs that whilst a listening ear and sympathy may be more valuable than hormone pills in the medical management of climacteric patients

> nevertheless, treatment of the physical symptoms of the menopause, hot flushes and sweats and atrophic vaginitis in particular, should be amenable to hormone therapy. Prevention of osteoporosis is important.
>
> (Coope 1987: 74)

Coope also stresses that any woman on HRT needs regular medical check-ups:

> during hormone therapy the patients should probably be seen every few months ... yearly pelvic examination ... is necessary ... yearly blood pressure check is useful and also weight and height measurement ... and a regular breast examination should be part of the follow-up. Women with a history of previous benign breast disease especially need surveillance on hormone therapy.
>
> (Coope 1987: 82)

Whilst *Women's Problems in General Practice* takes a relatively cautious approach to the use of HRT, other contemporary literature aimed at GPs is far more enthusiastic. For example, an article on 'Presentation of Menopausal Symptoms' written for a free magazine for general practitioners entitled *Well Woman Team* recommended treatment with HRT for menopausal women suffering from a range of vasomotor symptoms such as migraine-like head-aches and palpitations; older women suffering from 'aches and pains in the joints' or 'mood changes, irritability and depression, excessive tiredness and fatigue' and climacteric women suffering from more subtle forms of psycho-logical disturbances such as 'agoraphobia, panic attacks and loss of confidence' (Gangar and Key 1991: 8). Career women in their 40s who complain of 'loss of concentration and a general decline in mental faculties such as deterioration of memory and an inability to make decisions' should also be treated with HRT according to this article, despite the acknowledged lack of scientific evidence that these symptoms are menopausally related (Gangar and Key 1991: 9). Climacteric women suffering from a loss of libido or alternatively an increase in their sexual desire can, this article claims, be effectively restored to normal by the 'judicious use of HRT and testosterone'.

An editorial in the same edition of *Well Woman Team* argued that a conservative estimate would be that at least 40 per cent of climacteric women could benefit from HRT given for a period approaching five years. Although this might be costly 'more important than money, the quality of life of many women would have been immeasurably improved' (Stott 1991: 3). In particular the editorial emphasized the key role that HRT could play in preventing osteoporosis in elderly women. It suggested that one-third of all women – those who fall into the lowest quartile of bone density in either hip or spine – would benefit from taking HRT for five years after cessation of menses. This editorial also claimed that screening by bone densitometry to determine these at-risk women would be a cost effective management of the menopause (Stott 1991).

This new medical model of the menopause thus comprises two key elements. First, the immediate physical and psychological problems commonly associated with the climacteric are symptoms of a treatable deficiency disease. Second, an untreated menopause can and will create potentially lethal physical problems for women much later in life. The implications of this model of the menopause becoming universally accepted by the British medical profession and their older female patients are immense. Before this trend towards the universal treatment of the menopause with some form of hormone replacement therapy becomes unstoppable, women themselves should weigh up very carefully whether the claims made by the promoters of HRT are valid and whether the price older women may have to pay for this so called elixir of youth is too high.

HRT: an evaluation

There is plenty of clinical evidence to support the claim that HRT alleviates the physical problems of flushing and vaginal atrophy. For example, the American Medical Association stated authoritatively in 1983:

> An estimated 75% of women experience vasomotor flushes in the perimenopausal period or later ... Estrogen has a demonstrable and significant effect in reducing the intensity and the number of such episodes, or in eliminating them.
>
> (American Medical Association 1983: 359)

There is also the evidence of menopausal women themselves who have claimed that HRT has greatly relieved their hot flushes and completely solved the problem of vaginal atrophy (see Cooper 1979). Even here, however, there are some reasons for caution. First, clinical double blind trials have found that a placebo can be almost as effective in alleviating flushing as HRT (Coope 1987). Second, women who stop taking HRT after going through the menopause frequently experience withdrawal flushing (Coope 1987). Research suggests that only a *minority* of menopausal women experience severe physical symptoms (Coope 1987). Moreover, those women with relatively mild symptoms may find relief in simple non-medical remedies such as fresh air and gentle exercise or a change in diet – alcohol and coffee seem particularly linked to flushing (Reitz 1985).

Whilst even HRT's most vociferous critics do not suggest that it is ineffective in treating certain physical symptoms of the menopause, the claim that HRT can relieve psychological problems such as depression and anxiety is much less well supported by empirical evidence (see Ussher 1989). Indeed many medical experts do not accept that the climacteric as a physical event causes any noticeable psychological disturbances. If hormonal changes do not cause psychological problems, giving women hormonal treatment will be unlikely to solve their psychological distress unless it acts as a powerful placebo. There is some evidence that oestrogen given on its own helps some women to feel good, but in Britain very few women are prescribed unopposed oestrogen during the menopause. Most women are now given a mixture of oestrogen and progestogen which is somewhat similar – if much less powerful – to the combined oral contraceptive pill. Given that a well known side effect of the combined pill is 'increased irritation, anxiety and depression' (Berer 1989: 292) one can only puzzle at the logic of those experts who insist that in older women a very similar combination produces the opposite effect.

If it is more difficult than many women might suppose to find strong scientific evidence to back up the many claims for the immediate positive effects of HRT it is even harder to find conclusive evidence on HRT's longer term preventative role. Promoters of HRT stress that it actually saves many women's lives by protecting them from both heart disease and osteoporosis in later life. For example, according to Dr Peter Stott,

> Hormone replacement therapy given for five years at the time of the menopause can reduce the incidence of heart disease, stroke and osteoporosis, significantly lowering mortality and morbidity and improving quality of life.
>
> (Stott 1991: 2)

The claim that HRT could prevent heart disease in older women has been strongly pressed by the drugs companies. Wyeth Ayerst, for example, requested the US Food and Drug Administration (FDA) to allow the promotion of Premarin as protection against heart disease, at least for women who had had a hysterectomy. The FDA concluded that

> the cardiovascular benefits of estrogen replacement therapy with Premarin in women without a uterus may outweigh the risks, considering the individual patients' risk for various estrogen related diseases and conditions.
>
> (cited by Worcester and Whatley 1992: 18)

This somewhat cautious endorsement was reported in the popular press as 'benefits outweigh risks'. One enthusiastic promoter of HRT has even described it as 'terrific at protecting against heart disease' (Pike 1988: 70).

Such a claim is hardly warranted from the results of research into the relationship between taking HRT and the risk of heart disease. Whilst a number of research studies have reported a strong correlation between taking oestrogen during the climacteric and a lower risk of cardiovascular disease a number of experts are not at all convinced that this proves a causal relationship. The main issue is whether women who take HRT may be the type of women who are at lower risk of heart disease in any case. As an editorial in the *New England Journal of Medicine* pointed out in 1991, 'There is always the lingering possibility that women who choose to take postmenopausal estrogens have other characteristics that explain their lower risk of ischemic heart disease' (Goldman and Tosteson 1991: 801). Meanwhile, a review in *The Lancet* concluded that the epidemiological studies suggesting that oestrogen therapy prevents heart disease were fatally flawed (Vandenbroucke 1991). Another weakness in the link between HRT and low risk of heart disease is that this correlation has been found only in women taking oestrogen on its own. A number of experts strongly suspect that the addition of progestogens to oestrogen will negatively effect any potential benefits in relation to heart disease. For example, the *New England Journal of Medicine* cautioned

> Since added progestins reverse at least some of the favorable effects of estrogen on serum lipoprotein cholesterol, it is possible that the beneficial effect [of HRT on heart disease] is reduced when progestins are added.
>
> (Goldman and Tosteson 1991: 801)

Certainly it does seem odd that a combination of hormones very similar to those known to increase the risk of heart disease in young women is promoted as a protection against the same disease in older women.

By the early 1990s the most vociferous claim for HRT as preventative medicine was that it gave menopausal and post-menopausal women wonderful protection against osteoporosis. Most younger women had never heard of osteoporosis before articles in the popular press began to frighten them about it. According to the *Daily Express* (9 February 1993) for example,

> The most significant benefit of HRT is its role in preventing osteoporosis which can reduce the quality of post-menopausal life to almost zero and can, indirectly be the cause of death ... By the age of 80 half of all women will have had a fracture because of it. More depressingly of those who sustain a fractured hip, about a quarter will have died within a year and 50% will no longer be able to live independently.

After reading information such as that, it is hardly surprising that even symptomless menopausal women are keen to take HRT as a preventative measure. Moreover, even those who tend to be slightly anti-HRT have admitted 'there is considerable evidence of the beneficial effect of HRT on bone when given within 6 years of the menopause' (Phillips and Rakusen 1989: 470).

However, before more and more women are frightened into taking HRT primarily to prevent osteoporosis they should bear in mind the following three points. First, the drugs companies who manufacture HRT have conducted a very effective media campaign to ensure that fear of osteoporosis will boost sales. In the mid-1980s, following a dramatic drop in HRT prescribing in the US because of a scare over endometrial cancer, Wyeth Ayert, manufacturers of Premarin, hired a public relations firm to conduct a public education campaign aimed at encouraging all women over 35 to consider taking oestrogen to prevent osteoporosis. This campaign was a great success. In 1985 77 per cent of American women had never heard of osteoporosis, but by the end of the 1980s most women were worried that they might one day suffer from a severely bent spine or a potentially fatal fractured hip. The prescribing of HRT in the United States soared, from 15 million prescriptions in 1979/80 to 32 million in 1989. Premarin's annual sales which were valued at $400 million in 1989 were expected to exceed one billion dollars by 1995 (Worcester and Whatley 1992). Evidence of heavy promotion and high profits does not by itself indicate that HRT is not a safe and very effective preventative measure in relation to osteoporosis. Indeed, promoters of HRT claim that the costs of prescribing it will be greatly outweighed by the savings made in the treatment of osteoporosis and its consequences. There is, however, at least some significant doubt about the efficacy of HRT in preventing fractures in elderly women. In 1993 a study of 670 American women showed that HRT failed to preserve bone mass unless women took it for at least seven years, far longer than most British women take HRT. Moreover the study reported that even women who had taken HRT for 10 years or more had only 3.2 per cent higher bone density at age 75 than women who had never taken oestrogen (Felson *et al.* 1993). It thus appears that HRT may protect women from thinning bones when they are in their 50s, and not at great risk of fractures, but that this protective effect will not continue into old age unless women continue to take HRT for life. As an editorial in the *New England Journal of Medicine* commented, 'having to take estrogen for the rest of one's life reduces the appeal of this preventive strategy' (Ettinger and Grady 1993: 1192).

The appeal to women of this strategy – which involves them taking a powerful cocktail of hormones with a whole range of side effects for many years – might be further reduced if they were given unbiased information on other ways of reducing the risk of osteoporosis. For example, taking regular load-bearing exercise, as simple as walking briskly several times a week, can reduce the risk of osteoporosis. According to a review article in the *British Medical Journal* in 1992,

> selective use of oestrogen treatment will not provide an effective strategy for reducing the community's burden of osteoporosis. In contrast, regular exercise and stopping smoking are measures that most people can

aspire to and if adopted by the whole population may be expected to reduce the risk of hip fracture by 50% and 25% respectively.

(Jacobs and Loeffler 1992: 1407)

Unfortunately such preventative measures are non-profit making. Similarly, research has demonstrated that osteoporosis is by no means the only cause of serious fractures amongst elderly women. Falls in the elderly, for example, are significantly greater in women taking anti-depressants, sedatives and hypnotics which suggests that 'reducing rather than increasing drugs' could be the key to preventing the complications of osteoporosis in elderly women (Worcester and Whatley 1992: 11). Many falls in elderly women might also be prevented if all elderly women lived in good housing with adequate adaptations where necessary, but good housing for the poor has never featured highly on the health promotion industry's list of priorities.

Whilst more and more women are being persuaded to take HRT primarily to prevent osteoporosis in later life, many more are attracted to HRT by claims in the media that it will keep them looking young and beautiful. Younger women now talk about taking HRT in the same way as they weigh up the cost and benefits of a new miracle face cream. They tend to think of HRT in this way because of articles in women's magazines and the popular press with headings such as 'HRT – the drug therapy that can help a woman stay young' (*Daily Express*, 9 February 1993). They may also read quotations from medical experts who tell them that 'The point about oestrogen . . . is that it encourages collagen – a protein that makes bones, skin and hair strong and thick to form. (Studd 1988: 67). The idea that HRT prevents wrinkles, thinning hair and sagging breasts is a very seductive one in a culture which values women almost exclusively by their appearance, but scientific evidence that HRT improves women's looks is notable by its absence. One suspects that male scientists and male grant distributors are unwilling to waste their money and energies on such 'trivial' research yet drugs companies are by no means averse to implying that HRT can keep a woman 'feminine forever'. The problem for women is that HRT is not a cosmetic but a powerful combination of hormones. Given the known dangers of taking HRT long term many women may end up paying a very high price for their understandable pursuit of the holy grail of a youthful appearance in late/middle age.

The most worrying 'side effect' which any woman considering taking HRT needs to examine is the link between HRT and an increased risk of both endometrial and breast cancer. The first major scare in relation to the long term safety of HRT surfaced in the United States as long ago as the mid-1970s when the incidence of the diagnosis of endometrial cancer rose by 10 per cent. American doctors were so worried by the risk of women on HRT suing for damages if they developed endometrial cancer that they became very reluctant to continue to prescribe oestrogen-only menopausal therapy (see Worcester and Whatley 1992). In order to combat a very serious drop in sales the drugs companies developed and promoted a new form of HRT for women with intact uteri. They claimed that the addition of progestogens to natural oestrogen solved the problem of an increased risk of endometrial cancer by producing a withdrawal bleed which would ensure that a woman's endometrial cells were shed regularly. Unfortunately for women going through the climacteric – as Germaine Greer points out in *The Change* – the added progestins undo much of the 'feel good' factor associated with unopposed oestrogen. According to Greer 'progestogens make many women feel sicker than ever menopause did' (1992: 192). In any case, the adding of progestins to HRT has not eliminated the increased risk of endometrial cancer but only reduced it.

At least endometrial cancer is curable if diagnosed early enough, but there is now growing concern that HRT taken for a number of years increases a woman's risk of breast cancer, which is already very high. Promoters of HRT claim that the evidence on this is still not clear cut. According to John Studd, for example,

> There have been at least 25 papers on breast cancer and hormone therapy and none have been able to give startling figures ... Breast cancer is an age-related disease and extremely common. It is very hard to prove a definite link with oestrogen therapy.
>
> (Studd 1988: 67)

Yet several studies have clearly demonstrated a significantly increased risk of breast cancer in women who take HRT for several years. A prospective study of 23,000 Swedish women found an 80 per cent increase in the risk of breast cancer among women taking oestrogen on its own and a fourfold increase in risk among women taking oestrogen with progestin (Bergkvist *et al.* 1989). A review study published in 1991 reported a twofold increase in breast cancer in women, including some pre-menopausal women, who took combined HRT for 15 years or more (admittedly an exceptionally long time in the context of current British doctors' prescribing patterns). According to this study's authors, this increased risk would mean 4,708 extra new cases of breast cancer and 1,468 extra deaths in American women each year (figures based on 1987 US use of HRT therapy) (Steinberg *et al.* 1991). Whilst there is as yet no evidence to suggest that *short term* use of HRT significantly increases the risk of breast cancer, the existing evidence should at the very least make women somewhat wary of reassurances from HRT promoters such as 'If there was good evidence for a greatly increased risk, hormone replacement therapy wouldn't continue to be used' (Studd 1988). One presumes that neither the daughters of women who took Diethylstilboestrol or DES during pregnancy for threatened miscarriages nor the women who were injured by the Dalkon Shield would be terribly impressed by such an argument.

Some women suffering from severe menopausal symptoms may decide for themselves that an increased risk of cancer is a price worth paying for the immediate alleviation of their misery. They may then be surprised to find that far from making them feel wonderful, HRT may produce a wide range of unpleasant side effects. According to Kahn and Holt some of the most reported side effects from combined HRT are fluid retention, weight gain, breast tenderness, abdominal cramping, irritability, nausea and vomiting. They then go on to explain that more serious disadvantages can also occur. These include not only endometrial and breast cancer but high blood pressure, gall bladder disease and gallstones, abnormal blood clotting and jaundice (Kahn and Holt 1989: 98). Other sources outline other side effects until the list becomes almost endless. This does not mean that the cure is always worse than the original symptoms. Ecstatic endorsements of HRT from women whose lives were made a misery by severe menopausal symptoms, indicates that only some women taking HRT find that the 'cure' can be worse than the 'disease'. Nevertheless, the open acknowledgement by the medical establishment of so many possible negative side effects does at least suggest that HRT is by no means a panacea which should be automatically prescribed to virtually all women of a certain age. Those women who do experience distressing side effects from one type of HRT are sometimes advised by their doctors to take a different form of HRT. In response to the side effects produced by oral types of HRT, for example, many doctors changed to prescribing patches. Unfortunately a significant minority of women then experienced unpleasant side effects such as localized blistering with this method. An increasing number of doctors, therefore, turned to oestrogen implants but now it appears that up to 15 per cent of women taking HRT in this way actually become dependent on the oestrogen and need higher or more frequent doses of it to avoid unpleasant withdrawal symptoms such as hot flushes (Bewley and Bewley 1992).

Apart from questioning whether the risks to their health and well-being associated with all types of HRT may outweigh its benefits, older women might also like to consider carefully the extent to which the promotion of the menopause as a deficiency disease is leading to increased medical scrutiny and control over their lives. In the United States women prescribed HRT face a battery of routine tests and check-ups on at least an annual basis. It is common practice in the US, for example, to perform an endometrial biopsy annually on women taking HRT so that atypical endometrial hyperplasia and cancer can be quickly detected and treated (Coope 1987). Such an expensive and intrusive medicalization of the menopause has not yet been adopted by British doctors but clearly long term use of HRT does involve regular medical consultations and check-ups. One British gynaecologist who has run a specialist menopause clinic for many years has even suggested that postmenopausal women would be much better off having a hysterectomy followed by HRT than hanging on to their wombs.

Usually when women have a hysterectomy and then take oestrogen therapy alone, they say they haven't felt so well for years and wonder why they didn't have it before. There's every advantage in having the womb plus ovaries removed, and then having hormone therapy forever.

(Studd 1988: 68)

Perhaps older men might like to consider a similar option. Castration followed by long term testosterone treatment might quite rejuvenate them and would certainly prevent them from getting testicular cancer. But perhaps men would be less willing than female patients to accept such an extreme medical answer to their midlife crises.

One of the many consequences of the move towards a much greater medicalization of the menopause is that all women are now learning that at some point in their midlife they must face a major medical problem. At its most extreme the menopause as deficiency disease model paints a totally negative picture of the post-menopausal woman. According to Dr Robert Wilson

no woman can be sure of escaping the horror of this living decay. Every woman faces the threat of extreme suffering and incapacity ... Though the physical suffering from menopausal effects can be truly dreadful, what impresses me most tragically is the destruction of personality.

(Wilson 1966: 39)

Many medical supporters of HRT have disassociated themselves from the extreme rhetoric of Wilson's *Feminine Forever*. Nevertheless, the picture they paint of menopausal women who are not treated with HRT is hardly encouraging. Yet this increasingly negative medical picture of the menopause bears little relationship to what many menopausal women actually experience. Research has found that women who have actually experienced the menopause have, on the whole, much more positive attitudes towards it than younger women (Ussher 1989). Since younger women have no direct experience of the menopause whilst many older women still tend not to talk openly about this stigmatized life change, women's overall attitudes towards the menopause will inevitably be shaped by media images. The promotion within the media of the menopause as treatable deficiency disease model has clearly led to an upsurge in demand for HRT from older British women who are not being given nearly as much information on alternative, far less medicalized, approaches to this major life change.

The menopause can be viewed not as a medical problem but as a social and even a political issue. Paula Weideger, for example, in *Menstruation and Menopause* claimed that the greatest hazards of the menopause were culturally induced and would not be spirited away by a few pills. She cited a psychiatrist working in China who had never come across a menopausal psychosis in a Chinese woman which she attributed to the fact that in China the older woman had a secure and coveted position (Weideger 1976). In *The*

Psychology of the Female Body, Jane Ussher argued that in order to overcome women's understandable fears of the menopause

> we need to challenge the stereotypes which define women as useless when their reproductive function is ended. Ageist and sexist stereotypes in the media which reinforce the negative images of older women must be continuously criticised and challenged.
>
> (Ussher 1989: 132)

A key component of a feminist approach is to see not only older women but also the menopausal experience itself in a positive light. Reitz claims, for example, that her self-help approach to the menopause is potentially revolutionary because

> its emphasis is exactly the opposite to what we have been taught, consciously and unconsciously about our bodies. We have been taught to hate our bodies, hide our menstrual blood, fear our menopause and reject our aging. This book is about loving yourself, enjoying your body even relishing your hot flushes and embracing aging.
>
> (Reitz 1985: 1)

The New Our Bodies, Ourselves is less up-beat in its approach to the menopause but it too includes a positive emphasis and stresses that 'it is only a minority of women who experience problems that require medical treatment'. The book quotes one woman's very positive experience of the menopause:

> I welcomed the end of my menstrual periods because for years I had experienced premenstrual tension and heavy bleeding. The hot flushes were not a bad trade off if I could be free of periods at last. I have not had a period for four years. I feel healthier than ever, have an active and joyful sex life with no 'dry vagina' problems and do a lot of physical activities. This is definitely the best period of my life (a woman aged 51).
>
> (Phillips and Rakusen 1989: 456)

One way feminists suggest that older women can fight back against ageism combined with sexism in society is to meet together to discuss their experiences as older women. Support groups can not only increase women's understanding of the menopause and give them positive information and advice about it, they can also reduce individual menopausal women's sense of isolation and once again enable women to see personal problems as at least partially political issues. Writing in *Spare Rib* in 1983 Jean Shapiro suggested that women suffering from the emotional disturbances so commonly attributed to the menopause would do better to examine 'the pressures put upon her as a woman in a sexist and ageist society than simply rely on drugs of any sort' (Shapiro 1987: 66). She argued that a support group of older women could begin to consider the extent to which they have been pushed into expecting and adopting the stereotype of the unbalanced, depressed, ailing, inferior human being who is ill all the time and therefore useless.

Self-help groups can give women ways of coping with menopausal symptoms which avoid the need for medical treatment and supervision. A number of feminist oriented self-help books also now provide older women with a wide range of alternative approaches to reducing menopausal symptoms. They suggest, for example, that certain vitamins and herbal preparations may modify or reduce vasomotor symptoms such as hot flushes. Exercise has also been suggested as a way of reducing the frequency of hot flushes (see, for example, Phillips and Rakusen 1989).

At its most extreme a self-help non-medical approach to the menopause may run the risk of simply replacing one form of control and authoritarian advice by another. Not all climacteric women will wish to adopt the lifestyle advocated by Reitz, for example, who commands, 'You will certainly not eat cottony white bread or candy bars, for they are empty calories ... As part of loving yourself you'll read the printing on the yoghurt cups and you will buy only the natural ones' (Reitz 1985: 202). Such an approach tends to assume that all menopausal women are middle-class women with all the time and money required to devote themselves to a healthy lifestyle. Some older women may actually prefer to accept the advice and medical treatment of their GP than to follow a highly complex time-consuming and expensive self-help approach.

However by no means all non-medicalized approaches to the menopause are as didactic as Reitz's book. *The New Our Bodies, Ourselves,* for example, does not claim that alternative health can provide the answers to all women's menopausal problems. For some women HRT may well provide an acceptable solution to serious physical symptoms. The book simply points out that older women may like to explore a range of alternatives for themselves rather than simply to accept the medical model of the menopause as the only possible way through it (Phillips and Rakusen 1989).

Conclusion

It is perfectly logical to support the prescribing of HRT as a treatment for the more severe physical symptoms of the menopause whilst opposing its growing use as a panacea for all the problems women associate with ageing, including losing their looks. If HRT were to be routinely prescribed to most women going through the climacteric – whether or not they were experiencing disabling or distressing symptoms – not only would a significant amount of scarce health care resources be used up, but women would also experience further medicalization of their day-to-day lives. For a very small minority of menopausal women taking HRT over a number of years it could even prove fatal. Before being frightened into demanding HRT from their GPs – sometimes in advance of any menopausal signs or symptoms whatsoever – older women might like to pause to note the extent to which this demand for HRT is being created by the drugs companies. Whilst there does appear to be a significant body of medical opinion in Britain which genuinely believes that most older women would be better off on HRT than without it, women should never forget the very large profits to be made from the selling of HRT. By the early 1990s only around 10 per cent of menopausal women in Britain were being prescribed HRT at an annual cost of approximately £30 million (Stott 1991). Clearly drugs companies believe that the British market for HRT could still be expanded significantly. The means by which drugs companies promote HRT sometimes appear quite devious. In the mid-1970s Ayerst used a public relations company to plant articles on the menopause in American women's magazines and newspapers. These articles were to focus on the triumphs, tragedies and challenges of the menopause. To relay the 'estrogen message' discreet references would be made to 'products that your doctor may prescribe' (Lieberman 1977: 3). In Britain, drugs companies target much of their promotional activity at GPs. Whilst researching the menopause for this book I stumbled across a new free journal for GPs entitled *Well Woman Team*. Volume 1, number 4 featured two articles extolling the benefits of HRT. Both articles were written by medical experts but on perusing the small print I noticed that the journal was sponsored by CIBA Laboratories who just happened to have a full page advertisement for their hormone replacement therapy 'Estraderm' on the journal's back cover. Given the heavy involvement of drug companies in the development and promotion of HRT it is extremely difficult for even medical experts to assess the real risks and benefits of HRT. In 1985, for example, a doctor writing an editorial for the *New England Journal of Medicine* admitted

> I simply cannot tell from the present evidence whether these hormones [HRT] add to the risk of various cardio-vascular diseases, diminish the risk or leave it unchanged, and must resort to the investigator's great cop out – more research is needed.
>
> (Bailar 1985: 1081)

The danger is that no funding will be forthcoming for research studies into alternative approaches to the menopause. According to Germaine Greer there is even a danger that researchers in the not-too-distant future will not be able to find enough older women with intact uteri who have never taken any type of hormone treatment to act as research subjects or controls (Greer 1992).

Whilst drug companies have undoubtedly increased women's fears of the menopause through their promotion of this life event as a deficiency disease, they certainly cannot be held responsible for society's overall negative attitude towards ageing women. HRT may provide the medical profession with a powerful (and potentially dangerous) weapon with which to fight certain physical symptoms associated with the menopause, but even if HRT does slightly plump out the skin or thicken thinning hair, it cannot liberate older women from the combined negative impact of ageism, sexism and racism.

Older women are not greatly valued or admired by our society. Older men, on the other hand, can display grey hair, wrinkles and middle-aged spread without being written off as sexually 'past it' or mentally 'unstable'. Older men may be grey and even fat but as a group they are still powerful both economically and politically. If older women had similar access to economic and political power might not society begin to afford them more respect? Joan Collins, who extols the virtues of HRT, may look young for her age but we should not forget that she is also very rich and therefore powerful. HRT, far from transforming the lives of economically and politically weak older women, actually reinforces their fears of ageing. There will never be a miracle medical cure for the social and economic inequalities which stigmatize and marginalize healthy, attractive, competent women in their 50s. Older women as a group, therefore, need to ask some searching questions before taking at face value the promotional hype about yet another highly profitable drug which both benefits the drugs companies and increases the control which the medical profession already exercises over women's day-to-day lives.

5

MENTAL HEALTH CARE

It is widely accepted that women in the western world today suffer more mental illness than men, present psychiatric symptoms to doctors more often than men, and consume higher amounts of mental health care than men. The predominance of women amongst mental health care consumers is by no means a particularly modern phenomenon. During the nineteenth century large numbers of better-off British and American women were deemed by the male medical profession to be suffering from the uniquely female maladies of hysteria and neurasthenia. Doctors also ruled that women's reproductive systems not only weakened them physically but left them peculiarly vulnerable to mental and emotional disturbances. Any woman who took the dangerous step of thwarting her reproductive destiny or the even more dangerous step of damaging her reproductive system through over-educating and thus over-taxing her mind and body was deemed to be particularly at risk of going mad (Ussher 1991: Ch 4). Not only did nineteenth-century doctors define women as inherently mentally unstable, they also treated their problems with a range of physical and psychological treatments. Such 'cures' included clitoridectomy, ovariectomy (i.e. female castration) and a rest cure which comprised isolation, immobility and enforced feeding. According to Ussher this particular nineteenth-century cure closely resembled the modern torture technique of sensory deprivation which is applied to political prisoners (Ussher 1991: 75).

Late twentieth-century feminists have exposed these nineteenth-century treatments as a form of patriarchal social control. They have also pointed out that the medical treatment of female maladies such as hysteria was both highly profitable and prestigious (Ehrenreich and English 1979). Significantly, poor women were far less likely to be diagnosed as suffering from any form of female madness and less likely to receive any form of medical treatment – small compensation perhaps for all the other hardships endured by the Victorian poor.

Since the creation of the NHS, women in Britain no longer escape the medicalization of their lives solely on the grounds of poverty. Women are no longer diagnosed as suffering from hysteria or neurasthenia but far from dying out, the medical view of women as inherently vulnerable to most forms of psychological disturbance has continued to flourish and to affect more and more women's lives. As Ussher (1991) has pointed out, old fashioned diagnoses such as hysteria have simply been replaced by modern madnesses such as the premenstrual syndrome and postnatal depression. Women's biology, or more specifically their raging hormones, are still regarded by many doctors as key determinants of women's excess vulnerability to mental ill health. Women are also still perceived as the emotionally weaker sex by some doctors (see Roberts 1985). Whilst the contemporary medical model of mental illness does at least pay some attention to the role played by socioeconomic factors in the creation of mental health problems, most doctors still appear to believe that women suffering from more serious forms of depression, anxiety, phobias and baby blues are suffering from real physically based illnesses and are not simply reacting logically to intolerable circumstances (Rowe 1991). Not only are women still deemed by the medical profession to be inherently more vulnerable to mental disturbances at virtually every stage of their adult life from menarche to menopause and beyond, women are also still targeted as the main potential and actual consumers of a whole range of mental health care services. They consume more psychotropic drugs than men, more electroconvulsive therapy (ECT) and psychosurgery than men, more hospital treatment than men and last, but increasingly not least, much more psychotherapy and counselling than men, particularly in the private sector (Ussher 1991: 163).

In this chapter we will investigate women's experiences of mental health care services in terms of their effectiveness, their safety and their wider impact on women's lives. Before we proceed we should note that there will be very little discussion of the alternative explanations given for women's excess mental distress and no discussion of women's experiences of illnesses of a so-called psychotic nature such as schizophrenia. The main emphasis in this chapter will be on the treatment of depression and anxiety. We will begin at the beginning by looking at the impact on women of being given a diagnosis of a mental illness.

Diagnosis

The first stage in the medical treatment of women with psychological or emotional problems is usually diagnosis. Whilst the diagnosis of so-called serious mental disorders is primarily the domain of psychiatrists, in Britain, GPs diagnose and treat the majority of minor mental illnesses. Yet most practising GPs have received very little relevant formal training in the diagnosis and treatment of these illnesses. As one GP explained to Curran and Golombok

> We were trained by hospital doctors and the situation and problems are completely different. Hospital psychiatry really has very little relevance to general practice where we are dealing with emotional distress rather than psychiatric problems.
>
> (1985: 62)

Given their poor training it is hardly surprising if some GPs avoid a formal diagnosis when presented with a range of minor psychological symptoms and resort instead to a reassuring 'It's your age' or 'lots of women sometimes feel like this' before reaching for their prescription pads. Unfortunately the limited evidence we have of women's experiences of mental health care suggests that many women do not find such reassurances particularly helpful. In Agnes Miles's study, the women frequently alleged that their GP had minimized their complaint and lacked sympathy. One woman complained, for example,

> Dr D just said it was my age and the change. I told him I didn't think it was that because I still have periods. Then he said it could be the children leaving home, the nest emptying, but I told him my youngest son is only ten. He didn't want to know, just put me down as a nuisance. He is an efficient doctor but doesn't like nerve cases.
>
> (Miles 1988: 120)

Miles commented that

> Several women said that the doctors explained their troubles as 'usual women's problems' due variously to childbirth, menopause, menstruation or childlessness. It seemed to the women receiving such explanations, that inherent in them were dismissiveness and the trivialisation of their problems, which were regarded, by doctors as 'part of nature' or as 'over-reaction'.

If GPs fail to relieve their patients' distress by reassuring them and prescribing 'something to help their nerves' they may decide to refer them to a psychiatrist, on the grounds that psychiatrists are far more expert at both diagnosing and treating serious forms of mental distress. Women who are referred to a psychiatrist will usually receive an 'official' diagnosis based on one of the international 'bibles' of psychiatric diagnosis. The most widely used diagnostic manual is *The Diagnostic Statistical Manual of Mental Disorders* produced by the American Psychiatric Association (1987). This manual lists hundreds of specific psychiatric disorders such as dysthymia (or depressive neurosis), obsessive compulsive disorder (or obsessive compulsive neurosis), generalized anxiety disorder and post-traumatic stress disorder, to list but a very few. No doubt if a woman referred to a psychiatrist were to be shown this manual she would assume that such detailed, complex scientific knowledge was way beyond her own grasp. She might also assume that the diagnostic categories contained therein had the status of medical facts rather like the diagnoses of breast cancer or bronchitis. However a careful study of psychiatric textbooks and psychiatric journals soon reveals, even to the relatively untrained eye, that many psychiatric diagnoses are based more on educated guesswork or current fashion than on proven uncontested medical science. For example, one textbook of psychiatry begins by warning students that psychiatry is *not* a 'hard science' and that would-be psychiatrists must learn to live with uncertainty (Goldman 1992: 2). A good example of this uncertainty is the medical controversy over the division of depressions into reactive depressions and endogenous depressions. According to Storey's *An Introduction to Psychiatry* 'there are major disagreements among psychiatrists about this classification' (Storey 1986: 160). Yet many women are still told categorically that they are suffering from an endogenous depression for which there is no external cause. This is not always perceived as helpful or accurate by the patient:

> I was told I had an endogenous depression which I found out later was a depression that comes out of the blue and has no obvious cause. Well I felt the cause was obvious, I had plenty of explanations for it. But they just thought I was over-reacting I suppose.
>
> (Corob 1987: 11)

According to one leading British psychiatrist many doctors wrongly diagnose endogenous depression simply because they have not taken enough time or trouble to search for a relevant external cause of the patients' distress (Clare in Corob 1987: 11).

If psychiatrists frequently disagree amongst themselves about specific diagnostic categories of mental illness, such major uncertainty is very rarely conveyed to patients. But how useful is a clear psychiatric diagnosis to a woman suffering from acute mental distress? Limited research evidence and more anecdotal material strongly suggest that many women have found being diagnosed as suffering from a mental illness to be at the least unhelpful and, in certain cases, completely devastating. There are a number of clearly documented negative side effects of receiving a psychiatric diagnosis. First, and this is certainly not the fault of most psychiatrists, our society still imposes a stigma on the mentally ill. Thus even simply being referred to see a psychiatrist can have serious side effects on the patient. Friends, relations and work colleagues may, for example, react unsympathetically to such a referral. One woman in Miles's study, for example, reported that her husband reacted very negatively to her seeing a psychiatrist: 'Kevin is very unsympathetic ... He is sarcastic about psychiatrists. He says "I don't want a nutcase for a wife"' (Miles 1988: 103). A second problem experienced by some women who have received a diagnosis from a psychiatrist is that they simply have not understood it. This may leave them feeling stupid and/or confused. One woman in Miles's study reported, for example,

> I cannot understand what he is getting at ... he has his own way of saying things. If he could only explain better it would help ... When he starts explaining what depression is, I am lost and then I think I am stupid.

> (Miles 1988: 128)

A third and very significant side effect of a diagnosis from a psychiatrist is that a woman may feel as though she has now been labelled as mentally ill for life. One woman quoted by Alison Corob explained

> They told me I had a personality disorder and a clinical depression. This made me feel that there was something wrong with me that would never go away and that I would be labelled 'mental' for life. Really I think I was just very unhappy.

> (Corob 1987: 13)

In this particular case the patient had clearly resisted her diagnosis, but many patients who receive a diagnosis of a serious medical disease about which they have very little useful or understandable information may respond by feeling helpless and dependent on their doctor for effective treatment. If women are told by GPs and psychiatrists that their symptoms of anxiety and depression are undoubtedly caused by their hormones or by a genetic or biological 'fault' over which they have absolutely no control they are hardly likely to explore or change other aspects of themselves and their lives which may well be contributing to their extreme unhappiness. Yet Miles's research demonstrated that

> of all the factors which proved helpful to the women [who had received psychiatric treatment] who reported improvement or recovery, major events of the kind which brought about profound changes in their lives were the most important. These events included divorce or separation, moving house, relief from difficult caring roles and the obtainment of satisfactory employment.

> (1988: 145)

Naturally some women who are suffering extreme distress, for which they can find no logical explanation, may actually welcome a medical diagnosis which both explains the pain and relieves them of any responsibility for it. Our society may still attach a stigma to mental illness but an even greater stigma may be attached to bad behaviour, especially bad mothering, for which there is no medical explanation. One woman in Miles's study understandably felt greatly relieved when her poor mothering of her new baby was defined as 'postnatal depression' by a 'marvellous health visitor' (1988: 38). But the temporary gain of relief on being told that she is suffering from a genuine illness may yet be outweighed for many women thus diagnosed by the negative effects of the medical treatment which is then deemed necessary to 'cure' that illness. We will now examine the effects on women of the most commonly experienced forms of psychiatric treatments beginning with drug therapy.

Drug treatment

The great majority of women who are diagnosed as suffering from even relatively minor mental illnesses will be treated with drugs. There is nothing particularly new in this. During the nineteenth century hysterical female patients were given the sedative bromide. In the 1930s 'safer' barbiturates began to be prescribed and continued to be widely prescribed, despite growing evidence of their addictive nature and dangerous side effects, until the late 1960s when the benzodiazepines became available. By the 1970s prescriptions for tranquillizers and sleeping pills such as Librium, Valium, Mogadon and Mandrax soared and research demonstrated that women were twice as likely to be prescribed these drugs as men were (Ettorre 1992). In 1965 under five million prescriptions for Librium, Valium and Mogadon were dispensed. By 1979 30.7 million benzodiazepine prescriptions were dispensed (Gabe 1991: 4). During the 1970s, however, some doctors began to express concern over the misuse and overuse of these drugs and prescribing began to level off. The 1980s saw increased media concern over tranquillizer addiction and an actual decline in their overall prescribing. By 1991 'only' 19 million prescriptions of benzodiazepines were issued by GPs at a cost to the NHS of £19 million (Mental Health Foundation 1993: 25).

During the 1980s the main reduction in benzodiazepine prescribing was in new prescriptions as many doctors became more reluctant to prescribe tranquillizers and sleeping pills to anyone expressing relatively mild symptoms of stress and anxiety. Despite the very significant reduction in new prescribing, large numbers of patients are still long term users of benzodiazepine. By the late 1980s there were over one million long term users, two-thirds of whom were women (Gabe 1991: 5).

Before examining the major disadvantages of treating women's stress and anxiety with benzodiazepines we should note the good points about this group of drugs. First, they are relatively safe in terms of physical side effects, mental impairment and the risk of suicidal overdoses, compared to their predecessors, the bromides and barbiturates. Some medical experts still claim that Valium, for example, is a far less harmful drug than alcohol – the drug of choice for many stressed-out macho men (see Tyrer 1988). Mood altering substances have existed throughout history and in most cultures. Modern living is generally believed to be stressful. Doctors may be fully aware that what their patients really need is better housing or a job or a divorce but they cannot provide these stress relieving solutions for their patients, nor in many cases can their patients avoid the social conditions which may be creating their anxiety. If a single mother cannot afford alcohol to drown her sorrows why should she have to cope without any physical relief when mood lifting drugs are available on the NHS?

Whilst some doctors are now suggesting that the tide of opinion against the benzodiazepines has gone too far, some users of tranquillizers also object to the picture painted by 'tranx' opponents of women tranx users as helpless victims. Not all women who take or have taken tranquillizers are non-copers or helplessly dependent on their drugs. For some women the temporary and controlled use of tranquillizers clearly relieves unbearable symptoms and leaves them feeling more in control of their lives. For example, one woman in Miles's study claimed to take her tranquillizers only when she wanted to or felt she needed to: 'I know when I must take it but most of the time it's just there and gives me reassurance. I've managed to cut down but I still get the prescription in case I need more' (Miles 1988: 133). For women such as this a refusal to prescribe any further pills might well do more harm than good.

Whilst the media, and indeed some feminists, have tended to create a picture of a typical tranquillizer user as a young or middle-aged woman who uses the pills primarily as 'mother's little helpers', some research into long term users of benzodiazepines has found that long term users are now primarily elderly women who are suffering from poor physical health (Ashton and Golding 1989). It could be argued that elderly women who are in constant pain from complaints such as arthritis benefit from their use of hypnotics in terms of better sleep even if, as the critics claim, the effect of such pills after long term use is more placebo than real and even if they suffer some side effects from these drugs.

The fact that most people in acute distress, whether mental or physical, naturally seek whatever relief they can find from that pain, including in many cases drug-induced relief, does not mean however that drug companies and doctors have simply responded to innate consumer demand in producing and prescribing such large quantities of benzodiazepines. Nor does the fact that some women claim to have been 'helped' if not 'cured' through drug treatment for mental distress necessarily mean that such treatment has always been appropriate in terms of its undoubted benefits outweighing its costs.

Critics of the late twentieth-century tranquillizer boom have expressed a number of serious concerns over the relationship between profit seeking drug companies, doctors' prescribing habits and women in mental distress. First, the critics claim that benzodiazepines, far from being remarkably safe and side effect free, are both physically and psychologically addictive. Second, they argue that even the mildest of tranquillizers can produce disabling and/or unpleasant side effects. Third, critics suggest that tranquillizers are a form of patriarchal social control over women. Finally, some critics emphasize that both doctors and women themselves have been duped by the unethical promotion of tranquillizers by profit seeking drugs companies. We will now briefly explore each of these arguments in turn.

When the benzodiazepine drugs first became extensively available many doctors were extremely relieved to be able to give their distressed or sleepless patients a drug which claimed to be totally safe and non-addictive. One GP, for example, has written

> We welcomed them [tranquillizers] as replacing the barbiturates which were used by 4% of our patients. They clearly reduced the risk of successful suicide attempts. They also promised to cause less dependence.
>
> (Horder 1991: 165)

However, as early as the 1970s concern was growing within the medical profession that the benzodiazepines might not be quite the wonder drugs they had first appeared to be. Concern was expressed about both their real therapeutic value and their cost to the NHS. Then, during the 1980s, a new concern grew that the benzodiazepines could, after all, be addictive. Relatively small scale studies found, for example, that significant numbers of long term benzodiazepine users experienced withdrawal symptoms if they stopped taking them (see Ettorre 1992: 61). Accounts of withdrawal by individual long term 'tranx' users painted a harrowing picture of the withdrawal symptoms which some users may experience. One ex-user stated, for example,

> Frankly withdrawal has to be experienced to be believed. Vision is one of the first indicators – light is unbearable, faces distorted and hideous . . . You hallucinate. The backs of the eyes ache terribly . . . You find noise deafening. A light switch sounds like a bomb . . . I had choking feelings, palpitations, panic attacks, shaking, floating . . .
>
> (Maddocks 1987: 17)

Not only have women who have 'kicked' the tranquillizer habit described the awfulness of withdrawal symptoms, they have also described the 'deadening' effect which taking tranquillizers can create. One woman, for example, has contrasted how she felt whilst taking Valium with how she feels since she stopped taking it.

> I was on Valium for 15 years. Since I have been off I feel much better. I have confidence. I feel it is my own confidence. Before I knew it was only the pills which gave me confidence . . . For years I never used to notice the colour of the grass or the birds . . . When I was on the tablets I just used to go from day to day without noticing things around me. I feel that I wasted all those years on tablets. I never wanted to go out. Now I go out all the time . . . I feel alive again.
>
> (Curran and Golombok 1985: 98)

The majority of women in Miles's study mentioned drowsiness and tiredness which they ascribed to the drugs (tranquillizers and anti-depressants) which they were taking. A typical comment was 'I couldn't think straight, it's as though my mind was blocked off. I forgot everything I was so tired. When I stopped taking them I could think again. I was alert and I remembered things' (Miles 1988: 132).

For many critics of tranquillizers their most damaging side effect is not a directly physical one but the impact their use has on patients' abilities to think and feel their own way out of the situation which has caused their mental distress in the first place. According to Breggin minor tranquillizers are harmful in the long run not solely because they are habit forming and addictive but

> because they cover up anxiety by suppressing the capacity of the brain to generate feelings ... The drugged individual with a suppressed and confused anxiety signal system lives under a considerable handicap. At the least, feelings are pushed down and with that, self-awareness is muted.
>
> (Breggin 1993: 318)

This effect of tranquillizers needs to be considered in relation to what we know about the causes of women's anxiety and depression. Several studies have clearly demonstrated that women's vulnerability to anxiety and depression is closely related to their position in society and within their own families. For example, Brown and Harris's (1978) classic study of women and depression found that working-class women living in London were more likely to experience depression if they had three or more children under 14 living at home, they were unemployed, they had lost their mother in childhood or they lacked an intimate confiding relationship. In 1988 a study of women living on a south east London housing estate found that women diagnosed as depressed had much poorer marriages than a similar non-depressed group of women (Birtchnell 1988). Whilst GPs may be able to do little or nothing to prevent or alter very poor housing conditions or bad marriages, the prescribing of tranquillizers to women facing such problems must at the very least be regarded as a palliative for social inequalities rather than a cure for medical illnesses. Some critics of drug treatment go further and claim that doctors who prescribe tranquillizers to women suffering from male violence or the daily grind and isolation of unsupported motherhood are actually agents of patriarchal social control. According to Elizabeth Ettorre, for example,

> While these drugs may help her to 'stop making a fuss' about the contradictory feelings she is feeling as a woman, she is levelled out, unable to fight back and separated off from any positive forms of resistance. Rather than being empowered she is 'depowered'.
>
> (Ettorre, 1992, p 70)

Women's own accounts of tranquillizer prescribing and use clearly suggest that women have sometimes been prescribed drugs inappropriately in response to serious social problems. For example one woman in *Bottling It Up* reported, 'My husband was battering me and sexually assaulting me in front of the children. I told my doctor exactly what was happening and he told me to take Valium' (Curran and Golombok 1985: 35). Other women have explained how they take tranquillizers in order to fulfil their traditional 'caring' family role without becoming angry or aggressive. Cooperstock and Lennard's research based on group interviews with current and former tranquillizer users found that

> there were clear expressions of anger and resentment directed at their spouse by a number of women, at the same time as they saw no alternative to continued occupancy of the traditional wife, houseworker role'.
>
> (Cooperstock and Lennard 1986: 232)

We can conclude therefore that doctors do not have to be deliberately controlling their female patients' lives through benzodiazepine prescribing for such drugs to have a controlling effect. Women themselves sometimes use these drugs in order to control the anger and distress they experience at being trapped in oppressive circumstances. Moreover the male partners of some of these women clearly colluded in – and may even have initiated – this form of control. One woman in Cecil Helman's study of long term psychotropic drug users reported, for example, 'If I'm tensed up – my husband will say "Take a Librium"' (Helman 1986: 219). One woman took the concept of women taking tranquillizers in order to maintain 'happy families' and turned it on its head in a rather neat way:

> My husband was tense because there were problems at the office. His job was on the line for months and he was hell to live with. I told the doctor I was all nerves and got the Valium. I never took one, ever. I just put a pill in my husband's cup of tea every morning. It worked a treat. He still doesn't know to this day.
>
> (Curran and Golombok 1985: 50)

Critics of tranquillizers do not claim that their inappropriate use is solely the fault of the medical profession. They have also pointed out that these drugs have been aggressively marketed by the drugs industry. According to Ray (1991), 'Tranquillisers are the most profitable commodities in the world'. During the 1970s when Hoffman-la-Roche dominated the world market by producing 60 per cent of minor tranquillizers, their profit rate was 19 per cent – well above the average 5–6 per cent for manufacturing industries in OECD countries (Ray 1991). One of the key ways in which manufacturers such as Hoffman-la-Roche achieved such successful results was by the heavy advertising of tranquillizers to the medical profession. Research into the content of advertisements for psychotropic drugs placed in medical journals during the 1970s and 1980s consistently found that women featured in such advertisements far more than men. In 1984, for example, Melville reported that out of 115 drug advertisements for tranquillizers in the *British Medical Journal*, 91 referred directly to women patients (Melville 1984). In 1979 Chapman examined in detail five advertisements for mood altering drugs which featured women in stereotypical roles. Two of these advertisements featured house-wives and suggested that they would find routine household tasks less stressful if given the advertised drug. According to Chapman such ads might well appeal to a male doctor who might imagine that the woman depicted could be his own wife (Chapman 1979). Such advertisements thus reinforced doctors' stereo-typical views of women, their roles and their coping abilities. Many doctors understandably claim that they are not influenced by drugs companies' advertisements but research suggests otherwise. When Valium was advertised in medical journals more than any other prescription drug it became the most widely prescribed drug in the world (Prather 1991) thus confirming the efficacy of such advertising. During the 1980s advertisements for minor tranquillizers became much more gender neutral and tended to be based on abstract or neutral symbols such as a flower. Meanwhile however drugs companies switched their aggressive marketing away from tranquillizers towards new expensive types of anti-depressants. In the United States the new anti-depressant Prozac has been aggressively marketed and has become one of the most sought after anti-depressants of all time on the grounds that it not only lifts depression but leaves the patient feeling wonderful (Mauro 1994). Prozac is now being heavily advertised in Britain. According to a full page advertisement on the back cover of the March 1994 edition of the *British Journal of Psychiatry*, which was devoted to depression,

> Prozac matches the efficacy of tricyclic anti-depressants but not at the cost of impairing patient performance . . . And with its highly competitive price of £20.77 (for 30 capsules) Prozac is still cost wise the most economical SSRI you can prescribe.

Today, whilst many GPs are far more reluctant to prescribe benzodiazepines for 'everyday stress-related symptoms', they are happy to prescribe an anti-depressant for even quite mild forms of depression. In *Women's Problems in General Practice*, GPs are advised

> The majority of patients with major depressive illness respond predictably to anti-depressant medication provided it is given in adequate dosage and over sufficient time . . . Those with minor psychiatric disorders may also require temporary medication – a hypnotic if in crisis or a high state of arousal, or anti-depressants if a consistently low mood is described.
>
> (Greenwood 1987: 240)

In 1987 an article in the *British Journal of Psychiatry* even advised prescribing anti-depressants rather than benzodiazepines for persistent disabling anxiety symptoms that were not part of an adjustment or stress reaction. They also claimed that both acute panic attacks and agoraphobia responded better to anti-depressants than benzodiazepines (Tyrer and Murphy 1987).

Unlike the benzodiazepines, the anti-depressants have not been the subject of media criticism or general concern. Yet a few critics of the treatment of mental illness by drug therapy have claimed that, like benzodiazepines, anti-depressants are not only a very ineffective form of mental health care but are also dangerous, particularly if taken for any length of time. For example, Tricyclic anti-depressants can sometimes cause severe withdrawal symptoms and can therefore be addictive (see Breggin 1993).

Whilst in public, psychiatrists and GPs tend to reassure patients that anti-depressants are both effective and safe, when talking to each other a less optimistic picture is sometimes presented. For example an article in the *British Journal of Psychiatry* recently admitted

> Existing anti-depressants are unsatisfactory: they have limited efficacy, side effects are a problem and there is an appreciable degree of toxicity ... on any given treatment a significant number do not improve at all, while others improve at an unacceptably slow pace ... We cannot remain indifferent to the serious side effects of anti-depressants such as tricyclics.
>
> (Priest 1989: 7)

The author went on to illustrate the medical profession's continuing faith in drug treatment by looking forward to the wider use of a 'new class of anti-depressants' which he believed would have far fewer unpleasant or dangerous side effects (Priest 1989). These drugs would be a gentler version of the Monamine Oxidase Inhibitors (MAOIs) now commonly prescribed by doctors if tricyclic anti-depressants fail to work. It is reassuring that drug companies are attempting to create 'gentler' MAOIs since the current versions of these drugs are particularly unpleasant to take and particularly dangerous. When taking MAOIs patients must not eat a wide range of food and drinks in order to prevent severe and potentially life threatening cardiovascular reactions. MAOIs are also particularly lethal in overdose and 'withdrawal from MAOIs is more difficult than from tricyclics because the effects are likely to be more severe' (Lacey in Breggin 1993: 197).

Despite the many serious physical side effects and other major disadvantages of psychotropic drug treatment, for many women in an acute state of mental distress drugs appear to be the only answer. Unfortunately a large body of evidence now strongly suggests that the relief provided by psychotropic drugs is *at best* temporary and at worst bought at the cost of extremely disabling side effects. One woman cited in Corob's study nicely sums up the very limited benefits which psychotropic drug use provides:

> I've been on and off drugs – anti-depressants, tranx, for many years ... I think they help initially, maybe for a week or so, but then I think I'm only living to take another tablet. It doesn't solve anything, you still have to go back and face all the problems that were there before, but it perhaps helps you over a hump when life's really difficult and you can't handle it.
>
> (Corob 1987: 23)

Most women suffering from depression and anxiety will receive drug treatment whilst remaining in the community. A small minority of women with much more severe depressive symptoms will be hospitalized and limited evidence suggests that these women are likely to receive much higher doses of psychotropic drugs. In 1987 an article published in the *British Journal of Psychiatry* claimed that many severely depressed patients responded when the usual dose of tricyclic anti-depressants was increased to 200–300 milligrams daily. The article went on to present seven case studies (six women and only one man) of patients suffering from severe 'endogenous' depression who had proven resistant to lengthy trials of treatment with tricyclics and other anti-depressants. The author gave detailed accounts of the extremely high level of drugs prescribed to these patients. For example, Mrs AB was described as a 49-year-old woman with a unipolar depressive illness which had begun at the age of 44 shortly after a hysterectomy and salpingo-oophorectomy for endometriosis. Her father had committed suicide while depressed. On her second admission to psychiatric care following a serious suicide attempt her treatment included phenelzine (MAOI) 45 mg/day with trimipramine (tricyclic) 50 mg/day for one month, imipramine 150 mg/day and lithium 600 mg/day for two months followed by clomipramine 150 mg/day, tryptophan 2 g/day and lithium 600 mg/day (Hale *et al.* 1987). One does not have to be either a psychiatrist, or a pharmacologist to see that this is a lot of drugs. The authors of this article noted that doses of tricyclics had been increased for these patients until side effects were 'definite and moderate, but still tolerable'. In the cases reported this was usually at the onset of 'persistent postural hypotension'. They concluded that when patients failed to respond to very high doses of tricyclic anti-depressants a triple combination of lithium, clomipramine and trytophan should be tried 'before referral for psychosurgery' (Hale *et al.* 1987).

Where patients are a serious danger to themselves or others, the use of high doses of psychotropic drugs may be necessary but it must be noted that critics of psychiatric medicine have long been sceptical of such procedures and have emphasized how they may easily be misused to punish 'difficult' inmates of psychiatric institutions. For example, in her classic study of women and the American mental health care system, Phyllis Chesler (1972) claimed that women mental patients were frequently 'punished' for refusing to conform to society's stereotypical version of a good woman. Peter Breggin has even gone so far as to compare the situation of mental patients and battered women: 'Both the patient and the battered woman are most in danger of being treated violently when they reject being controlled and attempt to leave the hospital or the domestic relationship' (1993: 403).

Electroconvulsive therapy (ECT)

Whilst psychiatrists do not deny that drugs such as chlorpromazine are sometimes used primarily to control mental patients, most psychiatrists vehemently deny that ECT is also sometimes used as a form of control or punishment. They claim that this very negative view of ECT stems primarily from the film *One Flew Over the Cuckoo's Nest*, which is in no way an accurate portrayal of contemporary uses of ECT. Some psychiatrists appear both surprised and annoyed at the public's negative attitudes towards ECT. Peter Storey, for example, describes the campaign against ECT in the USA as 'strangely passionate and mainly outside the medical profession' (Storey 1986: 432) which is presumably intended to convey to medical students that they should not take the critics' case seriously. A number of psychiatric textbooks insist that ECT is both effective and harmless. For example, according to Goldman's *Review of General Psychiatry*, ECT 'is considered to be effective treatment for major depression' and

> modern techniques have significantly reduced morbidity and mortality [related to older forms of ECT] as well as allowing ECT to regain its place as a respected and legitimate method of treatment for selected patients with serious psychotic disturbances.
>
> (Goldman 1992: 388)

In Britain use of ECT appears to be in decline as psychiatrists put more faith in anti-depressant drug therapy, but in the year ending March 1990 more than 17,000 courses of ECT were still delivered (Breggin 1993: 228). It is clear, however, that women are still more likely to be prescribed ECT than men by a ratio of two or even three to one (Showalter 1987: 207). Critics of ECT claim that not only is it both ineffective and dangerous but its use is both ageist and sexist. We will examine each of these allegations briefly.

Controlled trials do not appear to have demonstrated that ECT has any positive effects on patients in the long term. For example, two British studies, in which real ECT was given to some patients and simulated ECT to others, found that the real ECT produced a significantly improved outcome after four weeks, but no significant benefit compared to the control group at six months (Buchan *et al.* 1992). In 1986 an American review of controlled trials of ECT concluded that no clear therapeutic effect of ECT in certain types of depression had been established (Breggin 1993: 256).

Advocates of ECT insist that the side effects it produces are usually minor and very short lived. According to Jack Dominian, for example, 'The only side effect following ECT is a memory disturbance that is short lived and leaves no enduring deficit' (Dominian 1990: 212) whilst Storey claims that patients who complain of long term memory loss after ECT are either likely to be 'people prone to obsessional ruminations', or people who 'have intellectual ambitions and interests which outrun their capacities. A course of ECT is then seen as the cause of their failure to achieve the success which eludes them. (Storey 1986: 433). In other words, according to Storey, patients who complain of long term memory loss after ECT should not be believed. Yet according to the critics of ECT it has been shown to produce long term memory loss in a significant number of cases. In one Scottish study 30 per cent of patients told their doctor that they felt that their memory had been permanently impaired (Freeman and Kendell 1986). One study of ten women following shock treatment reported that a number of the women actually thought that memory loss was the intended outcome of ECT. This study also implicated ECT as a form of patriarchal control. One woman felt 'the shock' was given to her specifically to make her forget her resentment towards her husband who had committed her to a mental hospital. Another woman's husband said of ECT, 'They did a good job there' because his wife's long term memory loss included a period when she had been in conflict with him. Three of the 10 women explained that they had lived in dread of ECT for years afterwards and had refrained from expressing anger towards their husbands for fear of being given more involuntary shock treatment (Warren cited by Breggin 1993). One doctor cited by Breggin had openly used ECT to reprogramme a woman's personality. A woman who had wanted to divorce her husband who beat her agreed to ECT after her husband threatened to get custody of their children. After ECT the woman (who changed her name from Peggy to Belinda) was deemed to be more 'balanced, more mature and adaptable in social situations . . .' Now, as Belinda her marriage is reasonably stable (Breggin 1993: 249).

In 1987 a supporter of ECT cited the case of a young female nurse who had suffered recurrent depressions 'brought on partly by her constant state of rebellion against authority'. After a course of ECT she 'led a normally turbulent life coping splendidly' (Romanis 1987: 55). Apparently it did not occur to her doctors to question whether her rebellion against authority might be perfectly justified in relation to a male dominated and authoritarian working environment. Whilst overt displays of patriarchal control and assault may be extremely rare amongst contemporary psychiatrists who advocate the use of ECT, even rare published accounts of ECT being used as a form of social control should at least give us pause for thought. We should also note that shock treatment is good business. One American psychiatrist admitted in 1977 for example that 'finding that the patient has [medical] insurance seemed like the most common indication for giving shock' (Breggin 1993: 235).

In Britain such a direct link between shock treatment and financial reward to doctors is far less obvious although there may be a danger that trust hospitals will begin to realize that psychiatric patients receiving 'shock' treatment could be more 'profitable' than those receiving other forms of treatment. However, even in Britain profits will be made from promoting and selling ECT machines. In the United States one professor of psychiatry who has been 'instrumental in bringing about the new trend of shocking elderly women' is actually president of a company manufacturing ECT machines and has admitted under questioning that he makes approximately 50 per cent of his income from Somatics Inc. (Breggin 1993: 237).

The trend for psychiatrists to recommend the increasing use of ECT on elderly women is one which must give rise to particular concern to all those who are not totally convinced of either the efficiency or the safety of such treatment. There is some very limited evidence that this trend is also occurring in Britain. A recent British audit of ECT in two NHS regions found that whilst some consultants used ECT 'sparingly when all else has failed or in life threatening situations' others regarded ECT as a safe and effective treatment for many with less severe depressive illness 'and *especially* in the elderly' (Pippard 1992; my emphasis). This study also noted that one psychogeriatric unit which was using 'an increasing amount of ECT' had totally inadequate recovery facilities.

Elderly women are particularly vulnerable to becoming psychiatric inpatients – not infrequently against their will. In 1986, 81 per cent of those aged 85 or over 'formally admitted' to psychiatric hospitals were women (Barnes and Maple 1992). Given the poverty, isolation and low esteem associated with elderly women it would hardly be surprising if they were particularly vulnerable to bouts of depression which is sometimes wrongly diagnosed as dementia (Barnes and Maple 1992). Is a course of ECT really the best solution to the complex range of problems faced by very elderly women in today's society? Or could it be that a course of ECT is simply a more cost effective and more capitalist compatible form of intervention than the provision of adequate income and social support which so many elderly women lack?

Behaviour modification

Whilst most women suffering from depression and anxiety are usually treated by the mainstream health care system with psychotropic drugs and much more rarely with ECT, young women with severe symptoms of anorexia nervosa may be hospitalized and subjected to a type of treatment known as behaviour modification. The key aim of this type of treatment is for the patient to make a rapid weight gain. Once a patient has achieved her target weight she is usually discharged from hospital as a 'successful' case although some patients may continue to receive out-patient care and counselling. Rapid weight gain is usually achieved within a hospital setting by a regime of behaviour modifi-cation which rewards (positively reinforces) the patient for any weight gained and punishes her (negatively reinforces) for any weight lost. Regimes vary from very strict to more lenient. In more traditional 'strict' regimes patients are initially confined to bed in a single room and are allowed no privileges until they have gained some weight. They cannot see relatives or friends and in some regimes they are not even allowed out of bed to use the lavatory. Every mouthful of food consumed is monitored and in some programmes patients are 'encouraged' to consume as many as 6,000 calories a day. Psychiatrists who pioneered this form of treatment in the early 1970s received enthusiastic support from the medical establishment (see, for example, Hussey 1974). Young women subjected to this type of treatment tell a rather different story.

Rosalind Caplin has recounted how she was hospitalized for anorexia nervosa during several of her teenage years. She describes her experiences thus:

> I was often imprisoned in a tiny room resembling a cell that had no access to daylight. I was robbed of basic human rights, such as using the lavatory or having a bath. I was psychologically as well as physically strait-jacketed and controlled in every sense of the word. When I could not – would not eat, I was force fed. It became the norm that every meal time I would be held down by two members of staff, one pinning my arms behind my chair while the other mechanically shovelled food into my mouth. The more this occurred the more I struggled until each meal became a literal battleground and I was left at the end with scratches all around my mouth and face and bruises upon my arms.
>
> (Caplin 1993: 11)

Another woman has described her similar treatment as 'dietary rape'. She described her experience of a behaviour modification regime as 'ceremonial degradation' and claims that

> the psychological damage it wreaked has long outlived even the pain of forced and coerced drugging . . . Punishment and reward programmes are merely brain-washing – punitive tortures which left me with no outlet for my distress.
>
> (Pembroke 1993: 20)

Not surprisingly patients' own criticisms of behaviour modification regimes are backed up by research data which show that for many anorexics weight gained whilst hospitalized is rapidly lost once they are discharged (Bruch 1974). Yet in 1992 the Court of Appeal ruled that a 16-year-old girl suffering from anorexia nervosa could be treated against her will at a unit for eating disorders in a London hospital. Lord Donaldson ruled that the girl's views carried 'no weight' in the decision on whether she should be treated (Dyer 1992: 76).

In many ways the use of strict behaviour modification programmes to treat young women hospitalized with the symptoms of severe anorexia nervosa can be held up as a paradigm of the patriarchal nature of women's experiences of the mental health care system. The patient is usually a very frail young woman. The consultant is usually a powerful man in charge of a medical team in which women very rarely have full equality of status and decision making power. The patient must behave in exactly the way prescribed by the medical staff. Such control may extend far beyond her eating behaviour. For example, one published treatment plan for a patient suffering from anorexia included in its list of short term goals for the patient, 'utilise cosmetics and accessories to enhance appearance. Be patient and wait my turn when delayed' (Levendusky and Dooley 1985: 217). In other words the patient must not only learn to eat properly, she must also learn to be feminine and submissive. One survivor of a behaviour modification programme for anorexia has recalled that

> sexist and heterosexist attitudes were common from the predominantly male white middle-class psychiatrists. Care with make-up and hair-style were seen to be clear indications of getting better, likewise wanting marriage and children were viewed by some as part of recovery. I know of individuals who have been told that their problem would get easier if they acquired a boyfriend.
>
> (Pembroke 1993: 21)

In recent years many hospitals have modified their programmes for treating patients suffering from anorexia and various forms of counselling and/or psychotherapy are now frequently included in treatment plans. Such modifications however do not necessarily alter the fundamental approach to anorexia adopted by hospital doctors nor do they change the essential imbalance of power between the patient and the hospital staff. One recent study of the treatment of anorexia included the case of a 17-year-old girl who was treated in a general hospital. At first she was confined to bed and gained weight rapidly. This initial weight gain was not sustained however and her case notes referred to her behaviour as 'very manipulative'. Her loss of weight resulted in her being fed by a naso-gastric tube whilst her psychotherapy became 'more intensive' (Monk 1990). It is rather hard to imagine this patient benefiting from psychotherapy whilst being force fed with a tube.

To be fair to psychiatrists attempting to treat women with severe anorexia nervosa, it is generally agreed to be a particularly difficult condition to treat and there is no clear evidence that counselling or psychotherapy by itself leads to any significant immediate weight gain. Given the real risk of patients dying from severe anorexia nervosa it is understandable if doctors attempt to exert some 'beneficial' control over their patients and thus over the disease itself. Unfortunately, the long term prognosis for those treated for anorexia nervosa is very mixed regardless of initial weight gain. Results from a range of follow-up studies of patients suffering from anorexia show that overall 40 to 50 per cent of anorexics do very well in maintaining a desirable body weight over several years. Twenty-five to 35 per cent have an intermediate outcome, 20 to 30 per cent a poor outcome and 4 to 10 per cent actually die from the disease (Guthrie 1990).

Many behavioural modification programmes only appear highly success-ful because patients are not followed up after discharge for more than a year. Even within the first year 'relapse occurs in about 50% of patients successfully treated in the hospital' (Hsu 1986: 578). It therefore appears that strict behaviour modification programmes which are clearly viewed as inhumane by many young women who have been subjected to them are not particularly successful in curing the disease they purport to treat.

Psychotherapy

Many critics of the current physical treatments for mental illness strongly advocate counselling or psychotherapy as a safer, more effective and more humane alternative. For example, according to Peter Breggin,

> Whilst psychotherapy, particularly Freudian psychoanalysis has abused women and men and will continue to do so, the talking therapies also have helped to liberate many women. Phyllis Chesler ... believes that many women have come to appreciate themselves and even to become feminists through psychotherapy. This is my experience as well.
>
> (1993:423)

Many women who have had very negative experiences of the various physical treatments for mental illness including drugs and ECT have demanded that medical staff should listen to them rather than treat them simply as a collection of medical symptoms. For example, a woman who was hospitalized several times with anorexia complained that her 'pain, grief and torment' her

> unexplored and unexpressed feelings were never addressed. When I was in tears, after eating a huge meal and feeling very scared, the nurse asked me to be quiet. I was told that they are not trained to counsel and hear how and what I was feeling.

After undergoing therapy this woman felt healed: 'I have surpassed my own expectations ... My insight has increased and I feel more capable of challenging the distress and disease that for so long has existed in me' (Neville-Lister 1993: 6). In Miles's study of women suffering from depression the consensus was

> don't take drugs and don't bottle it up ... if at all possible, one should find a sympathetic listener with whom to discuss problems. Opinions were divided on whether a professional or lay listener is to be preferred.
>
> (Miles 1988: 150)

In recent years there has been a massive increase in the availability of counselling and psychotherapy in Britain. Most of this expansion has occurred within the private sector where anyone, regardless of their qualifications or lack of them, can set themselves up as a counsellor or psychotherapist and charge clients significant sums of money for an hour of their time. Since this private sector is currently completely unregulated there are no statistics giving information on the gender of clients and therapists or the total amount of money now changing hands. It is clear, however, that the majority of private psychotherapy clients are women and that many are paying up to £50 a week for therapy which not infrequently lasts for several years. It is of course impossible to calculate or even begin to hypothesize about the effectiveness of such private treatment. Meanwhile despite opposition from a significant body of leading psychiatrists who continue to regard personal counselling as 'slushy, useless and crazy' (Child in Breggin 1993: 16), counselling and psychotherapy are becoming increasingly available within the NHS.

Whilst most critics of the bio-physical approach to mental illness put forward some form of talking therapy as a more effective person-centred alternative, some feminists have expressed serious concerns over the growing numbers of women undergoing counselling and/or psychotherapy. Feminists have pointed out that most of the talking therapies have been devised by men and are still controlled by men while most of their clients are women. Although in Britain a significant number of psychotherapists are female many of them have been trained within a system imbued with patriarchal values. Jane Ussher, for example, recalls that when she was working as a clinical psychologist her medical colleagues laughed at her for mentioning the feminist perspective on women's mental distress. 'No wonder' she writes, 'many women choose to follow the pattern in which they have been well trained, electing to practise the patriarchal therapies so expertly taught, to achieve a happy (and blind) progress up the career ladder' (Ussher 1991: 178). According to the more radical critics of psychotherapy even explicitly feminist therapists may convert women's structural oppression into personal neurosis. Kitzinger, for example, claims that feminist psychologists have contributed to the 'depoliticization of feminism by offering "personalised concepts to the feminist communities"' (Kitzinger in Ussher 1991).

Whilst even successful and non-abusive forms of therapy can be criticized for personalizing women's collective pain, critics of psychotherapists have expressed particular concern over the prevalence of sexual abuse within the therapeutic relationship. According to Ussher, studies attempting to investigate the issue of therapist–client sexual contact have indicated that up to 15 per cent of therapists admit to such activities (Ussher 1991: 180). Surveys of women clients who have been 'seduced' by their therapists have found that these women often felt they were to blame; they also usually expressed extreme distress after the abusive therapy relationship had ended (Schoener *et al.* 1984). Whilst representatives of psychotherapists may argue that those few therapists who sexually abuse their clients are a deviant minority who need special help, critics have claimed that they are more likely to be normal men exerting men's normal right to have a sexual relationship with a woman in a subordinate position. As Ussher has pointed out,

> These men are not an aberration. They do not behave in a way that deviates greatly from men in other positions in society ... sexual contact between powerful men and powerless women is part of the fabric of our society. Why should therapy be any different?
>
> (1991: 183)

Sexual abuse is not the only type of abuse which critics of psychotherapy claim may take place within the so-called therapeutic relationship. Jenny

Fasal, a private psychotherapist and the founder of an organization set up to combat abuse within therapy, has also called attention to the problem of addiction which she believes is widespread. She claims that if client dependence on a therapist is not recognized as a major problem vulnerable people can become addicted to their therapists and can end up in a worse emotional state than when they started (Fasal cited by Taylor 1992). Windy Dryden, Professor of Counselling at Goldsmiths College, has warned that some counsellors have a personal interest in keeping clients for as long a time as possible and that their motive need not be purely financial: 'Some therapists have the notion that the longer they keep their clients the better they are as therapists. They use this to bolster their self esteem' (Dryden cited by Taylor 1992). Whatever the motives of the therapist it is clear that women clients are particularly vulnerable to becoming very dependent on their therapists. One woman who became wholly dependent on a male clinical psychologist who then moved jobs has written, 'I felt I had been emotionally and mentally seduced. I loved him, in the end I would have believed him if he'd told me black was white' (Dryden cited by Taylor 1992).

Finally critics of the burgeoning psychotherapy industry have emphasized the profits and/or good living which therapists, counsellors and others can make from medicalizing women's distress. In an article on 'surviving the incest industry', for example, Louise Armstrong, herself a survivor of childhood sexual abuse, describes how an ever-growing sex abuse industry has medicalized what was originally a political issue.

> If our speaking out was an effort to litter the landscape with our cry for reform, they were the message suppressors, sent in by the powers that be, the sanitation engineers ... What they were after was medicalisation, making child rape an individual emotional problem (the child's). This not only de-issued the issue, it gave birth to a lucrative incest industry − counselling programmes, prevention programmes ... all of which was terrifically capitalism-compatible.
>
> (Armstrong, 1991, p 30)

Whilst many female clients who pay for therapy may argue that it is money well spent, growing evidence of abuse by male therapists of female clients must at least indicate that more research is needed into the safety and efficiency of the ever-widening range of talking therapies now being offered to women in distress. Without this evidence women cannot rest assured that they are not being exploited yet again by a medicalized treatment of their personal/collective problems.

Conclusion

Many health care providers who treat women who present with mental health problems are no doubt strongly motivated by a desire to relieve women of their distress. For example, one doctor quoted in *Bottling It Up* explained, 'It is nice to give Valium for a week to a patient who has just been bereaved to help her sleep and calm her down' (Curran and Golombok 1985: 70). Another GP admitted that gender played a role in doctors' treatment of women's mental and emotional problems:

> Most doctors are men, most patients are women. I have no doubt that there are some paternal, protective and sexual feelings between doctors and patients that make male doctors think they must help women more (than men). I think that women are also under far more stress than men basically in a sexist society.
>
> (Curran and Golombok 1985: 54)

GPs have also argued that lack of time may influence them to prescribe somewhat too many psychotropic drugs: 'You cannot always blame the doctor. The fact is the doctor has not always got the time' (Curran and Golombok 1985: 62). Finally GPs stress that since they cannot solve the socioeconomic problems faced by their patients they sometimes feel under great pressure to prescribe something to help their patients cope with that pressure (see Horder 1991). Despite all these reasonable arguments women can still object that the overprescribing of psychotropic drugs by GPs is ultimately de-empowering and reduces women's abilities to seek alternative, and in the long run, more effective remedies to their mental health problems. Moreover, whilst GPs themselves do not directly profit from treating women's mental distress, their status as valued professionals is enhanced by their role as experts in the treatment of minor mental illnesses. GPs may strongly deny that their treatment of minor mental illnesses is influenced by profit hungry drug companies but research has demonstrated how GPs' prescribing habits can be manipulated by forceful advertising (Prather 1991).

Women are clearly a 'prime market' (Ettorre 1992) for psychotropic drugs and whilst the drugs companies may have no direct interest in reinforcing women's traditional roles in society, the effect of their marketing their mood-altering drugs as the solution to the distress experienced by many women attempting to fulfil those roles has been to reinforce the individualization and medicalization of women's collective problems. The medicalization of women's distress sometimes takes an extreme form once women have been hospitalized. Women who become in-patients in psychiatric units are likely to be given very high doses of psychotropic drugs and if these have little effect they may be offered a course of ECT or even psychosurgery. One leading medical expert on the treatment of young women suffering from anorexia nervosa has used brain surgery as a last resort on intractable cases although he admits that 'the results are highly unpredictable' and that three patients are known to have committed suicide after a lobotomy (Hsu 1986).

One overall pattern which thus emerges from an analysis of the medical profession's treatment of women suffering from a wide range of mental illness is doctors' emphasis on physical treatments for what they regard as physically based illnesses. The dominant model of mental illness currently held by the great majority of British and American psychiatrists is that all serious mental illnesses have a biological or physical basis. For example, according to two American Professors of Psychiatry

> During the past 20 years ... a compelling body of information has accumulated indicating that many mood disorders (both severe and mild forms of depression and manic depression) are biological illnesses whose most effective treatment is medical. At present only psychiatrists are adequately equipped to diagnose and treat these depressive illnesses.
>
> (Rowe 1991: 333)

Without entering the very complex and sometimes acrimonious debate between those who see mental illnesses as primarily biologically determined and those who regard mental illnesses as primarily rational responses to intolerable stresses and strains we can at least note the element of professional self-interest in the above quotation. If women's problems are illnesses with very similar characteristics to physical illnesses then medically trained psychiatrists will be the profession with the expertise to treat their mental problems. If, on the other hand, women's mental illnesses were to be redefined as natural, logical even healthy responses to the varying stresses and extreme strains in their lives psychiatrists could conceivably be put out of business. According to Dorothy Rowe – a passionate critic of the biological approach to mental illness – psychiatrists the world over tend to favour a biological understanding of mental problems because if mental illness is

> simply a metaphor for the various ways we can feel despair, fear and alienation, the psychiatrists have nothing unique to offer. Anyone who has the necessary wisdom, sympathy and patience, a psychologist, a counsellor, a good friend – could give the help the sufferer needs. Psychiatry would vanish, just as the profession of hangman vanished from Britain once the death penalty was abolished.
>
> (Rowe in Breggin 1993: xx)

In Britain most psychiatrists are employed by the NHS and patients do not pay them directly for their services. This lack of direct payment tends to disguise the fact that psychiatrists are selling a particular service or product. They need to continue to attract customers or consumers of that product and the majority of their 'customers' are now – as they always have been – women. Linking this insight with women's own accounts of their experiences of the mental health care industry we can only conclude that it appears to provide far higher benefits for its employees and suppliers than it does for its main customers.

6

CANCER SCREENING

There can be few women left in Britain who remain totally unaware of either cervical smear testing or breast cancer screening. Most women aged between 20 and 64 will have received at least one written or verbal invitation from their GP to have a cervical smear test. Indeed some women may well have received many such invitations. Meanwhile most women aged between 50 and 64 should have received a written invitation to attend a local breast clinic for a mammography. According to the government these two national screening programmes will save many women's lives. In *The Health of the Nation* the government stated that

> successful screening (for breast cancer) detects the disease at a stage when there is scope for effective treatment. The aim of the programme is to reduce breast cancer deaths in the population invited for screening by 25% by 2000 compared to 1990.
>
> (Secretary of State for Health 1991: 65)

Given that breast cancer currently kills over 15,000 British women every year, 13,000 of them aged over 50 (Health Education Authority 1990: 6), such a goal must surely be welcomed by all women who understandably fear the high risk of developing this awful disease. Cervical cancer kills far fewer women annually, but according to the government many of the 1,700 annual deaths from this disease could be prevented if all women between the ages of 20 and 64 were screened at least once every five years in accordance with national policy (Secretary of State for Health 1991: 65). In this chapter we will first outline the dominant view of these two major cancer screening programmes. We will then present a minority view which claims that both cervical and breast cancer screening are inherently ineffective. The costs imposed on women who do attend for screening will then be assessed, including the costs imposed on women who receive medical treatment following a positive test result. Finally the relatively neglected issue of primary prevention of breast cancer and cervical cancer will be explored.

Cancer screening: the dominant view

In 1961 an article appeared in a leading American medical journal predicting the imminent demise of cervical cancer as a deadly disease (Lund 1961). The reason given for this extremely optimistic prediction was the introduction of the cervical smear test which, so the article claimed, would be accurate, inexpensive, widely applicable, acceptable to women and side effect free. The test would save lives because it would detect pre-cancerous changes to cervical cells which could then be treated before they developed into invasive cancer. In 1966 Britain began its own cervical screening programme. In 1965 only 700,000 smears were taken. By 1985 the figure was four million (McPherson and Savage 1987: 197). Deaths from cervical cancer, however, did not fall commensurately. In 1975 2,143 women died from cervical cancer, in 1985 the figure was 1,957 (McPherson and Savage 1987: 198) and by 1990 the death rate had fallen to about 1700 (Secretary of State for Health 1991: 65), but clearly the disease had not been totally prevented. Most medical experts and many feminist health care activists have claimed that the disappointing results of the cervical screening programme can be wholly explained by its mis-management and underfunding. For many years cervical screening was implemented in such a haphazard and unplanned way that women least at risk from cervical cancer were most likely to have a smear test whilst those most at risk – older working-class women – were least likely to be regularly screened. For example, a survey of over 600 women in the Tower Hamlets Health District carried out in 1985 found that 88 per cent of women aged 25 to 44 had had at least one smear compared to only 60 per cent of women over 55. Social class was also significantly correlated with whether or not women had had a smear, as 95.6 per cent of women in social classes I and II had had a smear compared to 77 per cent in classes IV and V (Savage et al. 1989).

One problem with the cervical screening programme frequently men-tioned in the medical literature during the 1980s was that opportunistic screening at antenatal and family planning clinics meant that many young middle-class women were over-screened, whilst the lack of a comprehensive screening programme based within general practice and the lack of good up-to-date practice records, particularly in inner city areas, meant that many older working-class women never even received an invitation to be screened. According to Alwyn Smith et al. Britain's screening resources were actually sufficient for regular coverage of the entire population but the fact that these resources were being concentrated on women with less than average risk of getting cervical cancer might well have been 'a major reason for Britain's lack of success in reducing the incidence of cancer' (Smith *et al.* 1989: 1663). Other critics have been far less sanguine about the adequacy of total resources for the British cervical screening programme. According to *The New Our Bodies, Ourselves*, for example, 'cervical screening is a political issue. Although it can prevent many unnecessary and premature deaths from cervical cancer the government refuses to fund an effective screening programme' (Phillips and Rakusen 1989: 530). Whilst many feminist health activists have campaigned for a better resourced and better planned cervical screening programme, popular women's magazines have also campaigned vigorously for more government action in this area. In 1992, for example, *New Woman* magazine told its readers that 'the screening programme is grossly underfunded. It is a situation that has angered many women who point out that the Government is allowing women to die whilst masquerading as their saviour' (*New Woman*, April 1992).

Not only has the government been accused of failing to ensure that enough women are screened regularly, it has also been accused of underfunding the laboratories which process the tests. Some laboratories have been so overwhelmed by demand, according to those calling for more resources, that their results have been far too inaccurate and some women have actually died quite unnecessarily as a result. In 1988 for example Brettony Mundy writing in *Spare Rib* claimed that many cervical screening laboratories had

> reached crisis point. They are understaffed and starved of essential funds and all the time and money spent encouraging women to have smears will ultimately be worthless if this appalling situation is not rectified.
>
> (Mundy 1988: 26)

For once most feminists and medical experts were united, more government money should urgently be put into the cervical screening programme in order to save women's lives. Some doctors however have also placed at least some of the blame for the failure of the cervical screening programme to date on women themselves. Whilst chiding some women for demanding too many smear tests, doctors have labelled other women as 'non-attenders' or 'non-compliant' and a great deal of medical energy has gone into trying to find out why such women resist something of such obvious benefit to them (see, for example, Beardow *et al.* 1989). Now that the government has introduced new incentive payments to ensure that GPs reach high cervical screening targets, some GPs are sounding increasingly angry with those women who fail to respond to their invitation to come in for a smear test. Discussions in the medical press have included the suggestion that once women have been identified as 'defaulters' they should have their notes clearly labelled to that effect. One practice however was prepared to 'excuse' and 'exclude' putative virgins whilst another was prepared to 'excuse' women who had been recently widowed (Ross 1989). In November 1990 *The Guardian* reported that one GP had even threatened to strike 20 women off his patient list on the grounds that their refusal to have a smear test was costing his practice £1,300 (*The Guardian*, 28 November 1990).

In summary, the dominant medical and lay view of Britain's cervical screening programme is that it is potentially a highly effective form of cancer prevention, but that it has failed to reach its potential, primarily because it has been badly organized and poorly resourced and second because some ignorant or wilful women simply refuse to use it properly.

The cervical screening programme was already seen to be running into serious difficulties when the government announced, just before the 1987 general election, that it was about to implement a national breast screening service. The government was responding to the recommendations of the Forrest Committee, which concluded in 1986 that the setting up of a national mammography screening programme for women aged 50–64 could save a third or more deaths from breast cancer (DHSS 1986). By 1990 77 screening centres had been established throughout England. The initial cost of setting up this very ambitious programme had been £55 million (Health Education Authority 1990: 7). The Forrest Committee based its claim of a 30 per cent reduction in mortality primarily on the results of two large randomized trials of mammography screening. The first, known as the HIP trial, took place in New York during the 1960s. In this trial women were screened by physical examination as well as by mammography and only 15 per cent of the cancers detected were found through mammography before they could be detected by palpation (see Skrabanek 1990: 628). Yet the results of this trial are frequently used to prove the efficacy of mammography screening alone. The other trial, known as the Two Counties Trial, was carried out in Sweden between 1977 and 1984. The Swedish researchers claimed a 30 per cent reduction in mortality from breast cancer in the group of women offered regular screening (who had a remarkably high 90 per cent attendance rate) (Tabar *et al.* 1988). In 1990 the results of a seven year randomized trial of mammography screening in the UK failed to replicate the results of the Swedish trial. The difference in mortality between the screened group and the control group after two years was not statistically significant (Roberts *et al.* 1990). Despite these very disappointing initial results older British women continued to be urged to accept mammography screening on the grounds that it could well save their lives. For example, a Health Education Authority leaflet entitled *NHS Breast Screening: The Facts* (1989) fails to give women the results of any of the large scale trials but concludes simplistically, 'When you receive an invitation to go for screening do accept. It's well worth it . . . Breast screening makes sense, it could save your life'.

Whilst urging women to take part in what can only be described as a mass experiment, some medical experts are already suggesting that if the British national screening programme fails to produce significant positive results it will be due – once again – to lack of adequate funding and even more crucially lack of compliance from women themselves. For example Ruth Warren, arguing the case for a national mammography screening programme claimed in 1988 that the Forrest Report's recommendations could only be implemented 'with difficulty, within the budget allocated' (Warren 1988: 970). In 1990 those responsible for the Edinburgh randomized trial of mammography screening blamed its initial lack of success on the fact that 'a large proportion of the study population' failed to attend for screening thus 'diluting any possible benefit of screening'. They concluded that 'A massive health education programme is required in the UK if attitudes are to change' (Roberts *et al.* 1990: 245). The researchers referred to comments made by the Swedish screening expert, Dr Bengt Lundgren who claimed that the negative attitudes of many women would jeopardize the success of the British screening programme. Lundgren blamed British women's 'ignorance', 'alienation', 'suspicion' and their 'largely ill founded lack of confidence in medicine' for their low compliance rate in cancer screening programmes (Lundgren 1988).

Cancer screening: the minority view

In order for any medical screening programme to be effective it must fulfil certain generally agreed criteria. The test must reliably distinguish those who do have an early form of the disease from those who do not. The disease must have a well understood and predictable natural history and finally and crucially there must be an effective available treatment which will either cure the disease or halt its progress (Skrabanek and McCormick 1989). A minority of medical experts have claimed that neither cervical screening nor breast cancer screening clearly meet all of these essential criteria.

Critics of cervical screening argue that the experts do not know enough about the relationship between minor abnormalities of the cervix and full blown cervical cancer to be able to claim that detecting the former prevents the latter. Current cervical screening techniques are detecting a very high level of minor abnormalities. Nearly 10 out of every 1000 women screened will have a positive smear of some kind (McPherson and Savage 1987), but it is now becoming much more widely accepted that a high proportion of minor abnormalities will not progress to invasive cancer even if left untreated indefinitely. McCormick claims, for example,

> The assumed benefit of [cervical] screening is largely based on the assumption that some abnormalities are precursors of invasive cancer, and that their identification and treatment will prevent serious disease. In fact, the natural history of these lesions is poorly understood, and furthermore invasive cancer may arise without evidence of progression through a series of precancerous stages.
>
> (McCormick 1989: 208)

In other words, many of those women who believe their lives have been saved by cervical screening would never have developed cancer in any case, whilst a few women screened at very regular intervals may nevertheless die of invasive cancer.

In order for a screening test to be effective it must not only detect a well understood progressive disease, the test must also be repeatable and reliable and thus able to produce consistent results, but McCormick claims, 'interpretation of smears has been shown to be very unreliable' (1989: 208). Moreover, as well as being intrinsically difficult to interpret many smears are 'technically unsatisfactory'. Dr Coleman cites the Head of Department of Cytology at a major London teaching hospital who reported that 10 per cent of all smears sent for analysis were useless and a further 40 per cent were of limited usefulness only (Coleman 1988). The main reason for this was that doctors had failed to take the smear correctly. Supporters of the screening programme have claimed that the current unreliability of laboratories is due to the fact that they are so underresourced and overworked, but the critics claim that even highly skilled experts find interpreting minor abnormalities very difficult and that this inherent problem inevitably leads to an unacceptably high rate of false positives as well as some false negatives (McCormick 1989).

If cervical screening has inherent weaknesses, and if the British programme has yet to demonstrate that it saves significant numbers of lives, why do so many experts insist that screening can and does work? Why have British women been told over and over again that cervical screening will protect them from cervical cancer? The evidence used to back this claim is usually taken from other countries. For example an article in *Spare Rib* in 1988 stated confidently

> In other countries substantial reductions in the mortality rate have been demonstrated – indeed in Sweden, Iceland and Finland the mortality rate has been cut by between 60–70% by using proper computer controlled programmes.
>
> (Mundy 1988: 25)

Such percentages are at first sight very impressive and persuasive but such statistics are not necessarily as clear cut as they seem. Peter Skrabanek, a most vociferous critic of screening programmes, has carefully examined the claim that those Scandinavian countries which have excellent screening programmes have significantly reduced mortality rates from cervical cancer whilst those countries without comprehensive screening programmes have not. Skrabanek (1987) claims that the argument that Norway has a much higher mortality rate from cervical cancer than Sweden because it has not had a proper screening programme is misleading. According to Skrabanek research has now demonstrated that 'from 1955 the cumulative mortality in Norway was decreasing at a slope similar to that in Sweden' (Skrabanek 1987: 1432). He also cites other countries such as Japan, France and Italy where mortality from cervical cancer is lower than in Sweden and has been falling for the past 20 years at rates similar to that in Sweden. Yet none of these countries has had nationwide screening programmes. Skrabanek concludes, 'The lack of correlation between screening activity and cervical cancer mortality is supported by a large volume of evidence' (1987: 1432).

Without being a highly trained statistician it is almost impossible for the lay reader to interpret and evaluate the very different conclusions which have been drawn from other countries' mortality rates from cervical screening and their correlation or lack of correlation with comprehensive screening programmes. However if one tentatively accepts Skrabanek's claim that screening programmes worldwide have had little impact on mortality rates from cervical cancer it becomes clearer that the lack of major success of the British screening programme may have less to do with its haphazard and underfunded implementation and far more to do with the intrinsic weaknesses of any cervical screening programme.

If the cervical screening programme is inherently weakened by the unreliability of the current smear test and the unpredictability of the disease itself, at least the early stages of cervical cancer can be successfully treated. Moreover, the declining mortality rate from cervical cancer does at least suggest that the national screening programme may be saving some women's lives each year. Critics of the national breast cancer screening programme, however, have emphasized that modern medicine cannot provide a similar cure even for very early breast tumours. In 1991 Sir Donald Acheson broke ranks with the majority of his profession when he admitted publicly that despite so-called advances in the treatment of breast cancer there had been no fall in breast cancer death rates throughout the 1980s and nothing more could be done in terms of treatment (Acheson 1991). This absolutely crucial point has become totally obscured in current debates over mammography screening, which focus almost exclusively on take-up rates and the major problems involved in reading mammography slides accurately. Very little is said in either the medical literature, or in the popular literature aimed at women, about how exactly doctors can cure the early tumours detected by mammography when they so patently fail to cure breast cancers detected by other means. Just before her own untimely death from breast cancer, Dr Maureen Roberts, once clinical director of the Edinburgh Breast Screening Project, wrote a very moving and honest critique of the very system she had helped to set up. In that critique she pointed out that doctors do not yet know how best to treat the small non-invasive tumours which will be detected by mass mammography screening programmes (Roberts 1989). Supporters of mammography screening constantly refer to the benefits of the early detection of breast cancers. Critics point out however that by the time a tumour is visible through mammography it will already have gone through 65 per cent of the time it would take to reach a size which could be detected through palpation. As Harold Hewitt has pointed out (Hewitt 1989) in order for mammography to be truly effective in actually reducing long term mortality from breast cancer it would have to be able to detect the majority of tumours before metastasis (spread) had occurred. But mammography, which only detects tumours which have already been growing for some time, could only prevent metastasis if dissemination of cancer cells only occurred relatively late in the history of the tumour. Hewitt concluded, 'This is distinctly improbable: if a tumour is capable of disseminating viable cells I see no reason why this capacity should be inhibited until a late stage in its history' (1989: 1337).

As we noted in relation to cervical cancer, in order for any type of screening to be truly effective the natural history of the disease being screened needs to be fully understood, yet scientists' knowledge of the natural progression of different types of breast cancer remains severely limited. What is now well known is that some very small tumours appear to be rapidly fatal, despite prompt discovery and treatment, whilst other much larger tumours are sometimes so latent or slow growing that they never prove fatal (Klemi *et al.* 1992). Given the different behaviour of similar looking breast lumps, choice of treatment following detection of such a lump through mammography is by no means straightforward. A lumpectomy or even a mastectomy designed to remove all cancerous tissue before it has spread will have no long term beneficial effect in those cases where metastasis has already occurred. On the other hand, some tumours excised by surgeons may never have spread dangerously in any case, and would not therefore have threatened the woman's life. In 1992 an article in the *British Medical Journal* concluded that

screen detected cancers were associated with features suggesting low levels of biological aggressiveness ... It is therefore possible that some of the cancers detected by screening might not surface during the lifetime of the woman and never threaten her life.

(Klemi *et al.* 1992)

The complexity of the natural history of breast cancers thus suggests that the promise made by the Health Education Authority and others that if symptoms of breast cancer 'are found at an early stage, there is a good chance of a successful recovery' (HEA 1989) is at the least simplistic. It certainly simplifies a very complex medical debate over the efficacy of medical treatment for so-called early breast tumours. According to one of the breast cancer screening programme's most vociferous critics, 'Thirteen out of 14 long-term follow-up studies of patients with breast cancer failed to show evidence of cure *regardless of the stage at diagnosis* (Skrabanek 1988b: 991). Similarly, Dr Maureen Roberts has emphasized within the medical press

We do not know how to treat breast cancer ... screening is not prevention ... the currently expressed or strongly implied statement that if women attend for screening everything will be all right is not acceptable.

(1989: 1154)

Breast cancer screening cannot prevent breast cancer, nor can it promise a cure; it is rather an attempt to gain better control over the disease. This simple truth has not got through to most women on the receiving end of mammography screening, mainly because the medical profession is reluctant to admit publicly that breast cancer has a low long term survival rate whenever and whatever treatment is given, and because British authorities continue to cite the 30 per cent reduction in deaths from breast cancer claimed by Swedish researchers. This percentage however may itself be a rather misleading way of presenting the results of the Swedish trial. According to Peter Skrabanek, 'The quoted 30% reduction is a relative percentage obfuscating the fact that the yearly benefit [of the Swedish trial] was one death fewer in each 15,000 women screened' (1988: 971). Even this figure obscures the fact that this small gain in relation to breast cancer was apparently offset by deaths from other cancers and other causes so that the overall mortality of the women in the Swedish trial was not reduced (Skrabanek 1988b: 971).

The way in which figures apparently indicating a significant benefit from screening may be presented to the general public in a misleading way is illustrated by Carolyn Faulder's *The Women's Cancer Book*. Faulder cites the results of a major UK trial of early detection of breast cancer. She describes its 20 per cent reduction in deaths in screened women as still counting as 'a significant improvement' (1989: 54). This ignores the crucial statement by the researchers themselves that a 20 per cent difference falls 'short of statistical significance' (Chamberlain *et al.* 1988: 411). In other words this small difference could have occurred by pure chance and did not prove in any way even minimal gains from the screening programme.

Negative side effects of screening

Health education literature strongly urges women to accept invitations for cancer screening, reassuring them that the tests involved are relatively simple and painless. Women are rarely informed of the great deal of evidence which has now been amassed documenting the harm many women have suffered following their participation in a cancer screening programme. First, there is evidence of the psychological distress women suffer when receiving what they believe to be a diagnosis of cancer. Current health education literature does at least try to reassure women that a positive cervical smear test does not mean that they already have cancer but it is clear that many women to date have failed to understand this crucial point. Women who have received the news that their smear test was 'abnormal' and that further investigation was necessary have frequently interpreted this news as a potential death sentence. One woman told Posner and Vessey, for example, that on receiving the news of an abnormal smear she 'planned her funeral', whilst another woman recalled that after being informed her smear test was 'positive', 'I lost half a stone in weight. I lost my appetite, felt sick. I had this awful feeling it was going to be cancer' (Posner and Vessey 1988: 45). Examples such as these demonstrate that the fear and emotional trauma that just receiving news of a positive smear test may cause women is in and by itself a major cost of the cervical screening programme. Further serious costs are then borne by all those women who go on to have further investigation by colposcopy (a magnifying glass with light) followed by medical treatment to remove any abnormal cervical cells. Standard treatments for cervical dysplasia now include out-patient procedures such as laser treatment or cryocautery which can be performed with a local anaesthetic or less frequently with no anaesthetic at all. Despite these new types of less invasive treatment however a number of women with 'pre-cancerous' abnormalities will still undergo a cone biopsy under general anaesthetic. One health education leaflet sponsored by Durex even suggests that after a positive smear a hysterectomy may be the treatment of choice for 'women who have completed their families'. However, even without under-going such an extreme form of treatment most women who are treated for abnormal cervical cells will experience physical, emotional and psychological side effects of varying degrees.

Physically, further investigation alone may be both humiliating and painful. The colposcopy examination has been described by some of those who have undergone it as 'unforgettable', 'distressing', 'unpleasant' and 'undignified' (Posner and Vessey 1988: 25). Eight per cent of women in Posner and Vessey's survey described the so-called painless examination as 'painful'. Out-patient treatment following investigation was experienced as painful by a much higher percentage of women. Thirty-eight per cent of women who had laser treatment said that it 'hurt, but not badly', while 44 per cent reported 'severe symptoms during treatment' and 38 per cent reported 'severe symptoms after treatment' (including physical and psychological distress). One woman described the pain during laser treatment as the worst pain she had ever experienced. Another woman who had been assured by the consultant that as the cervix contains few nerve endings it was relatively insensitive, reported that she was 'in agony' whilst undergoing laser treatment (Posner and Vessey 1988: 34–35). Despite the evidence of women's own experiences of severe pain, a straw poll carried out by *The Lancet* in 1989 found that only two-thirds of NHS patients were routinely given a local anaesthetic for laser treatment although interestingly *all* private patients received an anaesthetic (*The Lancet* 1989: 23). In reply to this editorial entitled 'Is laser treatment painful?', one obstetrician offering laser treatment wrote

> I was appalled to read . . . that laser treatment of the uterine cervix is done without anaesthesia. Treatment of the unanaesthetised cervix is always painful . . . I suspect that most laser therapists continue despite the protests

[from the traumatised patient] as they are all practising obstetricians and thus used to noise.

(Wright 1989: 335)

Apart from the immediate pain and emotional distress caused by the treatment of abnormal cervical cells, procedures such as laser surgery and cone biopsy do carry some longer term risks, such as the risk of an incompetent or narrowed cervix affecting a woman's ability to carry a pregnancy to full term (McTaggart 1991b). The extent to which routine treatment following a positive smear test may 'go wrong' is illustrated by an American case described by Robert Mendelson (Mendelson cited by McTaggart 1991b). A woman who was given a cone biopsy following a positive smear test bled so excessively following the operation that she was given an emergency hysterectomy during which she almost died from the anaesthesia; all this following the results of a test which is by no means a particularly accurate predictor of potential cancer in the first place.

Whilst a significant minority of women undergoing treatment following a positive smear test have reported significant physical side effects, even more women suffer psychological distress, not just because of the fear of cancer which the whole process almost inevitably provokes, but also because of the perceived association between cervical cancer and promiscuity. McCormick has suggested that because of the widely held belief that whereas nuns never get cervical cancer, prostitutes often do, women whose smear test proves positive have their characters as well as their cervices smeared (McCormick 1989: 208). Some women reported to Posner and Vessey that they strongly felt the stigma attached to having an abnormal smear. Several of the women had seen a TV programme which implied that only women who 'slept about' were at risk from cervical cancer. One woman said, 'I felt dirty because of the documentary on TV ... I was worried that everybody would think I'd been sleeping with everybody' (Posner and Vessey 1988: 67). Other women reported feeling defiled or unclean and several women reported that the positive smear test had adversely affected their sex life. For example, one woman explained, 'I felt my boyfriend wouldn't want to make love to me. I felt dirty and horrible' (Posner and Vessey 1988: 63). According to Jean Robinson, the widespread view that only promiscuous women are at risk from cervical cancer is a classic case of blaming the victim. She had met several women suffering from cervical cancer who had been firmly told by their gynaecologist that they should not have had sex with so many men. Yet as Jean Robinson has repeatedly tried to point out, a study as early as 1971 showed that if a woman had only one sexual partner herself but her husband was unfaithful her risk of cervical cancer increased (Robinson 1984).

Whilst the cervical screening programme clearly imposes heavy costs on some women who are screened, it does appear to offer the perhaps incalculable benefit of saving some women each year from a very premature death.

Unfortunately the cost–benefit ratio of the breast cancer screening programme appears to be even less advantageous to women coming forward for mammographies. Since the medical profession is still in no position to guarantee a cure to those women whose early breast cancer is correctly detected by mammography, some of these women will suffer many costs to very little benefit. For example some women will suffer from an increased length of time in which they must live with the knowledge that they have a life threatening cancer without being cured of the disease. As Skrabanek has pointed out, this knowledge 'may seriously affect the psychological well-being of patients' (1990: 629). Note how women who enter a screening programme as symptomless well women become 'patients' after receiving an initial positive result.

The psychological impact of a diagnosis of breast cancer – however early its stage – is known to be severe and in certain cases may even lead to major psychiatric illness (Lovestone and Fahy 1991). This psychological distress is likely to be acute whilst a woman waits for further investigation and possible treatment. Ironically by the early 1990s the national mammography screening programme had begun to detect so many possible cancers that women had to wait longer and longer for further diagnosis and actual treatment. One cancer specialist told the *Daily Mirror* in 1991 for example

> We are seeing increasing numbers of women with cancer which can be treated and cured. But we do not have the equipment to cope with them all. It is frustrating for doctors and very distressing for patients. But radiotherapy machines are very expensive and there is simply not enough money to buy sufficient of them.
>
> (Tong cited by Palmer 1991)

The implicit claim here is that radiotherapy can cure cancer, but the report of the consensus development conference on the treatment of primary breast cancer stated explicitly in 1986 'there is no evidence that radiotherapy prolongs life' although it can substantially reduce the risk of local recurrence of a breast tumour (Consensus Development Conference 1986: 946). The effect on patients of long delays before treatment for breast cancer commences can be illustrated using the words of one cancer patient who had to wait six weeks at a leading London hospital for radiotherapy for an inoperable tumour: 'I was in a total state of shock when they told me there was a six week delay, my mind was in such a whirl' (*Daily Mirror*, 25 September 1991).

Even if received promptly, the treatment for early breast cancer is often physically as well as psychologically traumatic. Whilst some surgeons and indeed some women may still choose a mastectomy as the 'safest' form of treatment for even the smallest of malignant tumours, the consensus medical treatment for early breast cancers has moved rapidly in recent years towards lumpectomy followed by radiotherapy and/or some kind of drug treatment. Whilst breast conserving forms of treatment are less disfiguring and disabling than mastectomies they are nevertheless invasive and not pain-free. Some women, for example, suffer serious pain and other side effects as a result of radiotherapy (Phillips and Rakusen 1989). Surprisingly there is little hard evidence to support the view that breast conserving techniques will reduce the psychiatric morbidity and sexual dysfunction known to be associated with mastectomies. According to an article in the *British Medical Journal* in 1990,

> There is still no evidence that breast conserving procedures ensure protection from psychological and sexual dysfunction. At least 13 studies which compared the psychological impact of mastectomy with that of lumpectomy found no overall psychological advantage to women who underwent breast conservation surgery. One study suggested that any advantage in terms of body image was offset by a greater fear of a recurrence of cancer.
>
> (Fallowfield *et al.* 1990: 575)

If the benefits to those women correctly diagnosed as suffering from breast cancer by mammography are far from clear cut, including the presumed benefit of being more likely to be offered breast conservation surgery, the costs to those women falsely diagnosed as possibly having breast cancer at first screening are already far too clear. In 1973 the American Cancer Society and the National Cancer Institute organized a massive nationwide mammography screening project. Four years later, following a controversy over its effectiveness, the National Cancer Institute appointed a committee of expert pathologists to review the tissue slides of 500 'minimal cancers' that the project had detected. These pathologists concluded that almost 10 per cent of those slides showed no evidence of cancer, but by that time 37 of those women had already undergone some form of mastectomy (National Institute of Health 1979).

The above is just one example of the very real dangers of overdiagnosis and treatment inherent in mammography screening programmes. In Britain specialists may well be more cautious in their treatment of 'minimal' cancers but the risks of false positive results remain high. Some experts have warned that the initial overdiagnosis rate in women screened by mammography may be as high as 30 per cent (Skrabanek 1988b). Even enthusiastic supporters of the national mammography programme have warned that unless a great deal of attention is paid to the advanced training of radiologists and centralized methods of quality control are developed and maintained, 'women will suffer unnecessary anxiety and unnecessary biopsies ... and the likelihood that lesions of dubious importance are regarded as cancer will increase' (Witcombe 1988: 910). Witcombe concluded that the undue haste with which the government was implementing a national screening programme would put healthy women 'at serious risk'.

Any woman who receives a recall letter after a mammography will experience a temporary diagnosis of possible breast cancer. In 1989 26 health authorities who had accumulated sufficient data for analysis presented a preliminary picture of the first results of the British mammography screening programme. Of those screened 7.4 per cent had been recalled for further assessment and 1.3 per cent underwent a biopsy. Of those biopsies approximately half resulted in a diagnosis of breast cancer. In absolute numbers this meant that over 8,000 women out of 164,000 had suffered the trauma of being recalled for further investigation, 1,410 had suffered the further trauma of undergoing a biopsy but only 733 women were ultimately diagnosed as having early breast cancer (Richards 1989). Using such figures it is not too difficult to work out the large number of women who will be put through the ordeal of further investigation following a single mammography screening once the national screening programme reaches its target of screening over three million women every three years. Even some of those who believe that such a programme will 'probably save some lives' have concluded, as usual in the relative privacy of the medical journals, that 'the number [saved] will not be enough to outweigh the damage to the women traumatised in the process' (Rodgers 1991: 1401).

Primary cancer prevention

Screening can be classified as a form of secondary prevention. It does not prevent individuals from developing the early stages or symptoms of a disease; it merely attempts to identify those symptoms in order to treat them before the disease they indicate becomes life threatening or disabling. Primary prevention on the other hand aims to prevent even the first stages of a disease or illness. Secondary prevention clearly fits well into a medicalized model of health and disease. It is carried out by trained medical personnel and tends to create more, rather than less, curative health care consumers. Secondary prevention is also marketable and profitable, particularly in fee-for-service medical care systems (Freeman 1991). Primary prevention on the other hand involves changing individuals' behaviour or changing social and environmental factors. Whilst health education can be medicalized and marketed to some extent, public health activity has not proved particularly interesting to most medical researchers and practitioners in the late twentieth century. In relation to cervical and breast cancer the medical profession's strong emphasis on secondary prevention through medicalized screening has distracted attention away from the primary causal factors in relation to these two diseases. A few medical experts, however, have begun to call for more research into the primary causes of cancer. For example, in 1991 after stating publicly that self-examination was not an effective method of preventing deaths from breast cancer, Sir Donald Acheson demanded urgent research into why so many women were getting breast cancer in Britain. He suggested 'I think the problem here is something to do with our general lifestyle and the way we live and what we do' (Acheson cited in Fuller 1991). In 1977 only one in 17 women developed breast cancer. By 1987 one woman in 12 could expect to develop breast cancer albeit with a marginally higher chance of surviving beyond five years (Faulder 1989). Researchers are pursuing a number of interesting possible causal factors for British women's very high risk of breast cancer including possible links between a high fat diet and/or a low fibre diet and an increased risk of breast cancer. Other researchers in Britain are attempting to continue and expand research which has already demonstrated that younger contraceptive pill users are significantly more likely to develop breast cancer in their early 30s than non-pill users (Chilvers *et al.* 1989). Yet despite this very worrying finding the government's medical research council withdrew its funding for further research in this area (possibly because of increased funding for AIDS research which kills far fewer women annually). A great deal of medical and epidemiological research is funded not by the government but by drugs companies. Understandably drugs companies are far more interested in funding research into treatments for breast cancer than into primary causes and preventive measures which would not involve the use of marketable drugs of any kind. Similarly, governments may be less than enthusiastic about funding long term research into relatively undramatic and complex issues such as the possible links between lifestyles, the environment and cancers, when they can make so much more political capital from funding much more highly visible and immediate projects such as the national breast screening pro-gramme. The same point also applies to the prevention of cervical cancer. The reason or reasons why some women develop abnormal cervical cells and some women go on to suffer from invasive cervical cancer are not yet fully understood by medical science. Some male researchers appear to have been obsessed with finding a causal link between women's sexual behaviour and cervical cancer. One American epidemiologist for example even purported to demonstrate in 1967 that patients with cervical cancer were seven times more likely to have first coitus on the ground than in bed (Rotkin cited in Skrabanek 1988a). According to Peter Skrabanek the links researchers, epidemiologists and doctors have constantly made between female promiscuity and cervical cancer are not only sexist and degrading but virtually meaningless, for as he points out, 'It seems that promiscuity, if it means anything, is having more sex than the investigator' (1988a: 579). Yet experts in the field continue to refer to the 'risky' sexual behaviour of young girls and continue, on the most part, to ignore the role of men in causing cervical cancer.

Epidemiologists' conviction that cervical cancer is caused by sexual activity has led researchers, at some time or other, to blame virtually every type of sexually transmitted organism known. For example, in the early 1980s the experts declared that exposure to herpes simplex virus type 2 could well be the causative factor in cervical cancer. Once that theory had been disproved the experts went on to blame the papilloma or genital warts virus. Women who are known to have been exposed to this virus are currently being advised by the experts to have annual smear tests or even colposcopy examinations. Yet according to an editorial in *The Lancet*, 'the high prevalence of papilloma virus infection in women with cytologically and colposcopally normal cervices casts further doubt on the oncogenic role of these viruses' (*The Lancet* 1987: 725). Indeed *The Lancet* editorial stated that whilst a wide range of sexually transmissible agents including spermatozoa, chlamydia trachomatis and herpes simplex virus type 2 have all come under medical suspicion at some time or other, 'proof of carcinogenesis has been lacking in every case' (*The Lancet* 1987: 725).

Lack of absolute proof of a sexually transmitted causal agent does not mean that women should ignore the strong likelihood that there is a link between penetrative sex and cervical dysplasia. Women should also be told that barrier methods of contraception should give at least some protection from cervical cancer. In one study 139 women with abnormal cervical cells were advised as their only 'treatment' to use condoms. In 136 women (98 per cent) their subsequent smear results went back to normal (Robinson 1984). If cervical cancer is sexually transmitted, men can clearly play a key role in preventing the spread of this disease. Yet despite the occasional reference in the press to 'promiscuous men' causing cancer, the government and the medical profession have placed all their preventive emphasis on screening and virtually none on the simple primary prevention method of barrier contraceptives such as the condom.

Whilst most researchers have emphasized the links between sexual activity and cervical cancer far fewer have emphasized the links between age, social class and cervical cancer. No other cancer has in fact such a steep class gradient, with women in social class V being four times more likely to die from cervical cancer than women in class I (Davey 1988: 30). One possible explanation of this strong association is that working-class women are more likely to be smokers than women in class I and smoking appears to increase women's risk of developing cervical cancer (McPherson and Savage 1987). Another possible risk factor which has received least attention of all, however, is the role of industrial pollutants to which working-class women's husbands are much more likely to be exposed. In 1981 Jean Robinson produced evidence of a clear link between husbands' 'dirty jobs' and their wives' cervical cancer. Her research was more or less ignored, but in 1987 the Office of Population Censuses and Surveys (OPCS) confirmed a clear association between a high risk of cervical cancer and manual work, notably metal workers and building labourers. According to Robinson,

> The typical victim [of cervical cancer] is not a bright young career girl who had fun and is now paying for it, but an elderly woman who lived for much of her life in a house without a bathroom and was married to a man who came home in dirty overalls.
>
> (Robinson 1981: 16)

Given the popular and misleading view of cervical cancer as a disease suffered primarily by the promiscuous, it hardly seems surprising if older monogamous women married to men in 'dirty' manual occupations fail to perceive themselves as at risk and therefore as needing a smear test. Even more significantly the general lack of interest in the link between industrial pollutants and cervical cancer allows industrialists to continue to provide poor protection from industrial pollutants in factories and other workplaces. The cost of cleaning up men's working conditions could well prove far in excess of the millions of pounds now poured, so far rather ineffectively, into the national cervical screening programme.

Discussion

Whereas primary prevention is usually unprofitable, and may even significantly reduce industry's profits if it involves reducing environmental pollutants or the manufacture of harmful products such as cigarettes, medical screening can be both profitable, prestigious and politically advantageous. Manufacturers of medical equipment, for example, are keen to expand the use of mammography machines. Medical supply companies, for example, now advertise mobile mammographic units. According to Medical X-Ray Supplies Limited

> regular early warning health screening facilities ... should be the entitlement of every woman, and with this intention Rollalong and Medical X-Ray have combined their expertise to design a mobile mammography unit.

The rapid expansion of mammography screening in Britain however probably has less to do with profits and more to do with politics and the priorities of medical scientists. The Forrest Committee's Report was published just before a general election and Dr Maureen Roberts has claimed that the government's very positive response to it was a 'political decision' (Roberts 1989). Dr Roberts pointed out that whilst the government was quite prepared to put a relatively large amount of resources into a national breast screening programme of unproven value, it was not prepared to take any serious measures which would harm the tobacco industry, despite overwhelming evidence that any reduction in cigarette smoking could save thousands of lives each year from lung cancer and many other diseases. In 1992 John Major told the readers of *New Woman* magazine

> We were the first country in the EC and one of the first in the world to introduce a computerised cervical and breast screening call and recall

system and the new GP contract encourages GPs to give higher priority to health promotion services for women.

(*New Woman*, April 1992)

Clearly women's health has become a political issue but debates about the efficacy of mass screening programmes have been kept out of the political arena.

Politicians' acceptance of mass screening programmes is partly a case of following doctors' orders. Doctors themselves may well be attracted by the national mammography programme because, as Dr Roberts has pointed out, it 'seems prestigious', but she continues

> it is possibly in danger of becoming a highly technological service. There is also an air of evangelism, few people questioning what is actually being done. Are we brainwashing ourselves into thinking that we are making a dramatic impact on a serious disease before we brainwash the public?
>
> (Roberts 1989: 1154)

Many of those running the new mammography centres are actively involved in research. According to one researcher the national breast screening programme 'creates an unrivalled opportunity' to compare results which have been obtained in different ways from different screening centres. Not only will researchers be able to study the effects of different screening and recall systems but

> The programme may have spin-offs too. The screening population is a captive one, which makes it possible to record additional information on family history, for example, in a uniform way on a very large scale.
>
> (Stewart 1988: 51)

In other words women attending for mammography screening are unwittingly taking part, yet again, in medical research.

Whilst the cervical screening programme in Britain has been less well organized as a research programme it too now provides significant income and profits to large numbers of people, and has also been seen as a political imperative. McCormick has suggested that cervical screening was originally hailed with great enthusiasm by the medical profession because gynaecologists found it so hard to watch women, some of them young, die in pain from a cancer which was theoretically curable if detected and treated early enough. According to McCormick, 'There was no question of randomised controlled trials because the results would speak for themselves' (McCormick 1989: 209). When such results failed to materialize, rather than questioning the test *per se*, experts blamed the poor results on the 'fact' that those women most at risk were failing to come forward to be screened. Meanwhile screening rapidly became 'politically popular' and many women, accepting the doctors' insistence that a comprehensive screening programme could save many women's lives, blamed politicians for not spending enough on cervical screening.

Governments responded to what was for once united pressure from both medical experts and women themselves and significant sums of money were soon being given to both a national screening programme and new 'high tech' forms of treatment for those women whose smear tests proved positive. Interestingly, whilst feminist health care activists have been quick to note the dubious motives behind the pushing of elixirs such as HRT, they appear to have paid little attention to the ulterior motives behind mass screening programmes. Yet in one sense cervical screening could now be seen as a major industry in its own right, employing large numbers of people both directly and indirectly, and offering a rewarding career to those at the top of the screening tree and at the forefront of experimental ways of treating women 'suffering' from abnormal cervical cells. The type of gross profit making associated with, for example, the widespread prescribing of Valium to women is clearly absent in preventative medicine, but not only do some medical experts make their names in such programmes, but GPs now have very explicit financial incentives to screen virtually every adult woman in their practices including the reluctant ones. These incentives have led to a significant change in tone and emphasis within the cervical screening programme. Whereas in its early days women very much had to opt *in* to screening, many GPs are rapidly moving towards a recall system designed to allow only a few women in very specific categories to opt *out* of being screened. They are also resorting to invitation techniques which include sending women a birthday card offering a 'well woman check as a birthday present from the practice' (Chomet and Chomet 1990). Major financial incentives for GPs to be pro-screening are hardly likely to encourage the screening agnostic or atheist to stand up and be counted amongst those who see little or no benefits in the programme. Finally and not wholly facetiously we should note that someone somewhere is probably making a tidy profit out of the basic equipment – such as all those glass slides needed to take and then analyse millions of smears annually.

Given the small but undoubtedly real risk that some cases of mild cervical dysplasia do, if left completely untreated, progress eventually to full blown cervical cancer, it is very hard to suggest to any woman that she ignores all invitations to have a smear test. Given that the test itself is relatively painless and quick, many, if not most women, who fully understand the nature and purpose of the test will probably decide that their individual cost-benefit analysis leads them towards rather than away from screening. This does not mean, however, that it is in women's interests as a group to be pushed into a near compulsory screening programme. In 1989 James McCormick argued that

> screening for carcinoma of the cervix by cervical smears satisfies none of the criteria which would provide its justification. It is an expensive contribution to ill health because the harm exceeds the possible benefits by a substantial margin.
>
> (1989: 207)

The cervical screening enthusiasts have yet to prove McCormick wrong. Whilst cervical screening in Britain developed in an extremely haphazard and unplanned way, the national breast cancer screening programme was very carefully planned from the start in order to avoid the known problems of cervical screening. Unfortunately good planning alone cannot ensure medical effectiveness. Whilst the possibility that mammography screening may save some lives cannot yet be ruled out, it is already clear that claims that a third of all deaths from breast cancer could be prevented are, at the very least, optimistic. Ironically a report in the *British Medical Journal* on the programme results for 1991–92 claimed that it could be regarded as 'extremely satisfactory' on the grounds of a high acceptance rate of 71.3 per cent and a low referral rate for further investigation of 6.2 per cent (Chamberlain *et al*. 1993). What the report failed to mention was whether any of this activity would actually prolong or save the lives of women detected as having early breast cancers. Satisfactory referral and detection rates are hardly enough in themselves to justify the massive financial and emotional costs of a national screening programme.

Despite all the known drawbacks of Britain's experimental breast screening programme, including the rarely emphasized pain and discomfort which significant numbers of women experience whilst having their breasts squeezed between the two metal plates used to x-ray them (see Rutter *et al*. 1992), older women may still decide that on balance mammography is beneficial to them on the grounds that a tumour detected through mammography should be more treatable by the most conservative means than a more advanced tumour. For this benefit to be of real value to women however, it is essential that resources are provided for caring and comprehensive treatment programmes as well as for the more high tech aspects of cancer screening and subsequent treatment. Women diagnosed as suffering from breast cancer need good psychological as well as good physical treatment. Some cancer specialists are beginning to accept a more holistic approach to the treatment of women with breast cancer, others remain vehemently opposed to all forms of so-called 'alternative' treatment. It is clear, however, that a cancer treatment programme which provides ample support and counselling for each individual patient will be more costly than a programme which simply conveys patients along a high tech production line. In 1986 a consensus conference on the treatment of breast cancer stated that each health district's breast cancer service should include the services of a trained nurse counsellor. In 1989 Dr Maureen Roberts made a moving plea for more research into the psychological aspects of breast cancer treatment and suggested that

New psychological methods designed to improve the quality of life (and indeed not impossibly quantity of life) – for example self growth and visualisation, as well as more conventional approaches – should all be considered.

(Roberts 1989: 1155)

Apart from demanding cancer treatments which will provide universally high standards of psychological and emotional care as well as effective physical treatments, women must continue to resist the view that medicalized cancer screening equals cancer prevention. Those seduced by the optimistic claims of cancer screening enthusiasts might do well to recall the sadly misplaced enthusiasm in the 1960s for x-ray screening for early lung cancer. Eventually attempts to reduce deaths from lung cancer turned away from totally ineffective early detection to primary prevention in the form of anti-smoking campaigns, albeit with no real support from successive governments which were benefitting from tobacco tax revenues. It seems highly likely that women will have to wait until the causes of breast cancer are better understood before a new primary prevention strategy will begin to have a real impact on Britain's extremely high incidence of breast cancer. Unfortunately the experts seem far more excited at the prospect of a new type of screening programme in relation to breast cancer than in any primary prevention research. Geneticists now claim that they are close to identifying a gene which causes familial breast cancer and already one US company has been set up to market a genetic screening test which would identify women at high risk from breast cancer. What options would a young woman testing positive in this new genetic test face in terms of preventing breast cancer? According to an article in the *New Scientist* in 1993 one possible option would be 'prophylactic surgery – an anodyne clinical term that means removal of both breasts and possibly both ovaries' (Brown 1993). Even this drastic option could not eliminate all risk. Another alternative would be for a young woman at risk to take the drug Tamoxifen – a drug known to have a number of unpleasant side effects and feared to have potentially dangerous long term effects (see McTaggart 1993). Many women may find the very idea of prophylactic double mastectomies appalling but geneticists are already warning that as soon as a genetic test for breast cancer is available 'there will be a commercial interest attached to seeing as many people screened as possible' (Brown 1993: 37).

The imminent commercial development of a genetic screening test to identify women at very high risk of developing breast cancer suggests that once again a form of medicalized screening is going to dominate cancer prevention strategy. Whilst many of those who provide cervical and breast screening services undoubtedly believe that such services benefit the women who use them, the one-sided promotion of these services clearly disguises their inherent weaknesses. Women faced with increasingly heavy handed attempts to pull them into medicalized screening programmes of any kind should therefore try to maintain a healthy scepticism. Cancer screening programmes provide a whole range of benefits to all those involved in providing them. There is, as yet however, no conclusive proof that these programmes provide enough benefits to those women pulled into them to outweigh their well-documented physical and emotional costs.

7

HEALTH PROMOTION

Radical critics of the NHS have claimed that far from being a health service, it actually focuses almost exclusively on ill health and disease. Priority has consistently been given to the 'high tech' acute health care sector which, so the critics claim, has failed to cure far more often than 'miracle' success stories in the media lead the general public to believe. Critics of high technology medicine have often called for a major shift in emphasis within the health service away from acute hospitals and towards primary prevention and health promotion (e.g. Garner 1979). By the early 1990s health policy makers finally appeared to be taking on board at least some aspects of such a change in emphasis. In 1991 the government's consultative document *The Health of the Nation* heralded a new strategy, 'to improve the span of healthy life' primarily by focusing 'as much on the promotion of good health and the prevention of disease as on treatment, care and rehabilitation' (Secretary of State for Health 1991: vii). Health promotion had finally won a powerful seal of approval, but central government's version of health promotion very much emphasized the responsibility of individuals to adopt healthy lifestyles rather than adopting a much more structural approach to the creation and maintenance of a healthy population. Many women would agree with the government that they should protect their health by giving up smoking, drinking less alcohol, eating better and exercising more – even if they find it much harder to put such a healthy lifestyle into practice. Women also worry about the unhealthy habits of their families – will their children eventually die from heart disease if they continue to eat beefburgers and chips for lunch rather than steamed fish and vegetables? Will their husbands have a heart attack if they eat butter rather than margarine? These are certainly the type of worrying messages which women are receiving from an ever-expanding health promotion industry, but how scientifically valid are all these official pronouncements on a healthy lifestyle? Are women as wives, mothers and above all mothers-to-be really primarily responsible for the health of the nation? In this chapter we will examine three key areas of the current health promotion strategy – smoking, alcohol and diet. Three key themes will emerge from our analysis: first, the scientific accuracy or rather inaccuracy of the health education messages given to women; second, the extent to which such messages exert oppressive social control over women's lives; third, the inability of the health promotion industry to tackle the primary causes of women's unhealthy behaviours and health problems. We will begin by examining the government's strategy to reduce smoking amongst women.

Women and smoking

The setting of official national targets for reducing cigarette smoking amongst women outlined in *The Health of the Nation* might be regarded as somewhat belated given the long history of women's smoking in Britain and its long-standing appalling effects on women's health. British women began to smoke in significant numbers during the 1930s when cigarette manufacturers first began to target women specifically in their advertising. By 1939 women were smoking approximately 500 cigarettes per head per year. During the Second World War cigarette consumption per head increased fourfold among women in the UK compared to only one and a half times amongst men. By the late 1950s female smoking reached a peak at 44 per cent of all women. This figure did not begin to decline in any sustained way until the mid-1970s (Jacobson 1988). From then on women did begin to quit smoking in significant numbers but at a slower rate than men – many of whom incidentally took up pipes or cigars instead. By the early 1990s 30 per cent of all adult women still smoked compared to 33 per cent of all men, but this small difference in percentages was mainly accounted for by more men than women smoking over the age of 60. At younger ages the figures are now remarkably similar. For example in 1988 28 per cent of girls aged 16–19 smoked compared to 28 per cent of boys (Secretary of State for Health 1991: 67).

The evidence that smoking is directly responsible for very high levels of excess morbidity and mortality among women is undisputed. By the late 1980s over 10,000 women per annum were dying of lung cancer in England and Wales and the great majority of these deaths could be directly attributed to smoking. This death toll is the equivalent of killing all the women in a small town every year (Charlton 1990). In Scotland the death rate from lung cancer amongst women is even higher and has now surpassed the annual death rate from breast cancer. In fact Scotland now has the highest lung cancer rate among women in the whole of Europe (Charlton 1990). Lung cancer, of course, is not the only life threatening disease closely associated with cigarette smoking. Many thousands of women die each year from heart and respiratory diseases which are smoking related. Smoking also increases the risk of women developing other cancers such as cancer of the larynx. Several studies have also suggested that women who smoke are at increased risk of cervical cancer. Finally it is well known, and particularly well publicized by health experts, that smoking during pregnancy is associated with low birth weight babies. Smoking also increases the risk of a wide range of complications during pregnancy and labour (White 1987).

When government funded health education campaigns against smoking were first launched in the 1960s, women simply did not feature. It was as though cigarette smoking was solely a problem for men. It was not until the early 1970s that women began to appear in anti-smoking campaigns. For example the Health Education Council featured a character called Fag Ash Lil in a TV commercial and the British Medical Association advised women to give up smoking in order to prevent premature wrinkles (!) (Jacobson 1981: 70). When health promoters finally began to take women's smoking more seriously they typically focused on the harm smoking caused not to women themselves but to unborn fetuses. In 1973 a major anti-smoking campaign was launched featuring a poster of a nude pregnant woman with the caption 'Is it fair to force your baby to smoke cigarettes?' An accompanying TV commercial showed a tiny baby lying in an incubator whilst a voiceover warned, 'You may deprive your baby of oxygen . . . you may poison its bloodstream with nicotine . . . it may even threaten his life' (Jacobson 1981: 71).

This very frightening form of health education certainly made pregnant women smokers feel more guilty and anxious about the harm they were told they were inflicting on their unborn babies but there is no evidence that this type of campaign actually reduced smoking amongst pregnant women. Yet many health experts continue to assume that lecturing pregnant women on the harm smoking may cause to their babies will have a positive effect. Health policy makers also continue to prioritize the need to reduce smoking amongst pregnant women rather than seeing all women smokers as important in their own right. For example in *The Health of the Nation* central government's only specific commitment of extra resources to fight its anti-smoking battle was a £1 million grant to the Health Education Authority to carry out a project 'to provide information and support to women to enable them to stop smoking during pregnancy' (Secretary of State for Health 1991: 67).

Traditionally doctors and other health activists have tended to assume that women who continue to smoke during pregnancy are either ignorant or irresponsible. They have therefore concentrated their efforts on informing, sometimes aggressively, pregnant women of the dangers of smoking. More recently, however, some researchers and health promoters have begun to point out that this individualistic model of smoking during pregnancy is too simplistic and ultimately ineffective.

According to research by Ann Oakley (1989) some anti-smoking pro-grammes aimed specifically at pregnant women, particularly those offering good support at the local level, have achieved some success in enabling a mi-nority of pregnant smokers to quit. However, many pregnant women continue to smoke throughout pregnancy despite being all too aware of the health hazards involved and despite sometimes almost constant nagging and lecturing from antenatal staff – why? Oakley suggests that pregnant women who experi-ence a lot of stress in their lives, including the stresses involved in pregnancy itself, may find it impossible to give up or cut down on their smoking despite being fully aware that they ought to do so. One woman in Oakley's study of mainly disadvantaged pregnant women described, for example, how her re-lationship with the baby's father had ended during her pregnancy. She had then taken an overdose of paracetamol and had been admitted to hospital. She had promised the clinic doctor that she would try to cut down on her smoking but told the researcher, 'I tried to give up but I get so I want to kill everybody. I don't think it's worth it at the moment. I'd have to get right away. From every-one' (Oakley 1989: 325). Oakley concluded her study that pregnant women continue to smoke 'as a defence against environmental circumstances that are themselves hazardous to health' (1989: 330). Oakley also queried why doctors and other health experts focus so strongly on smoking as a health hazard during pregnancy when epidemiological studies have suggested that other factors such as diet may play a significant role in determining, for example, babies' birth weights. She comments, 'Perhaps diet being more obviously de-termined by income is less clearly a matter of individuals choosing to be un-healthy?' (Oakley 1989: 330) Research has also suggested that the link between smoking and low birth weight babies is significantly modified by social class (Rantakallio cited by Oakley 1989: 263). Yet in *The Health of the Nation* the government again emphasized the link between maternal smoking and low birth weight and mortality without any mention of social class or, in particular, material deprivation as a key risk factor during pregnancy and childbirth.

Whilst pregnant women have been targeted by specific anti-smoking cam-paigns since the early 1970s it was not until the 1980s following the publication of Bobbie Jacobson's *The Ladykillers* that British women health activists began to put effective pressure on male dominated health promotion bodies such as the Health Education Council (HEC) and Action on Smoking and Health (ASH) to devote more of their resources to the problem of women smokers in general. During the 1980s anti-smoking campaigns and action programmes designed specifically for women multiplied at the local level – most notably in Scotland – and in 1991 central government's *The Health of the Nation* lent support to local initiatives to reduce the proportion of women who smoke by setting specific 'realistic' targets for all health care providers to aim for by the year 2000. Health experts have, on the whole, welcomed this new initiative but critics have argued that, despite the rhetoric, central government's apparent commitment to reducing rates of smoking in both men and women is seriously undermined by its complete failure to commit itself to an outright ban on all cigarette advertising. An article in *The Lancet*, for example, commented

> Despite the success of 20 states that have introduced advertising bans on tobacco, the Government decided to continue with its voluntary code – a code so unsuccessful that the industry is recruiting 450 new young smokers a day to replace the 100,000 plus it kills every year at the other end of the life cycle. The unhealthiest link of all, of course, is the industry's links with the Conservative Party. In the last election the tobacco industry gave the Conservatives 2,000 prime advertising sites to promote their campaign. Now it has been well rewarded.
>
> (Dean 1992: 166)

Dr Anne Charlton's research into the factors influencing smoking in girls and boys aged 12 and 13 found that awareness of cigarette brands and positive views on the effects of smoking (for example that it will calm nerves, look grown up, give confidence and control weight) were among the most significant influential factors for girls whereas for boys having a best friend who smoked was the most related and positive beliefs the least related of any influence analysed. Charlton's research also demonstrated that advertising presented the message to young women and girls that 'smoking takes away your fears and stress and moves you into a magic world' (Charlton 1990: 32). If they had a favourite cigarette advertisement 32 per cent of 9 and 10-year-old girls who had never smoked believed that smoking calmed your nerves. Of those who did not name a favourite only 16 per cent believed it. In recent years cigarette advertisers have been severely restricted in the types of message they are allowed to put across through advertising. Due to these restrictions some brands are now advertised through surreal posters with no clear cut message at all. Such restrictions have not, however, stopped manufacturers influencing young girls' smoking behaviour. One 15-year-old girl interviewed by Jacobson who had recently started smoking Benson and Hedges said their ad was her favourite: 'It's such a good ad, it really impresses me. I'd like to hang a picture of it in my bedroom' (Jacobson, 1988: 71). Not only are young girls very aware of cigarette manufacturers' poster campaigns, they are also still exposed to advertisements in magazines, despite the voluntary restrictions which ban advertising in magazines at least a third of whose readership is aged between 15 and 24. Amos *et al.* have demonstrated that the voluntary restrictions introduced in 1986 had failed to protect young women and girls from cigarette advertising in magazines. For example *Bella*, which does not come under the restrictions because it is read predominantly by older women, nevertheless had about 924,000 readers aged 15 to 24 (i.e. about 22 per cent of all British young women of that age group). Moreover the voluntary agreement did not even cover style magazines such as *The Face, I-D* and *Blitz* which are particularly influential among contemporary young readers (Amos *et al.* 1991).

Not only are children and young women influenced by a range of direct forms of cigarette advertising, they are also being exposed to various forms of sponsorship and promotion by tobacco companies. Perhaps the most notorious example of such promotion was Martina Navratilova's outfit worn at Wimbledon in 1982 which bore the distinctive logo and colours of Kim cigarettes, a brand which had just been launched in the south east of England with a major advertising campaign aimed directly at young women. More recently tobacco companies have moved into the world of rock and pop music which they see as 'the key to the youth market'. According to *Campaign* (a magazine for the advertisement industry), rock stars are after all 'blank billboards waiting for brand names to be attached' (Jacobson 1988). Some British record companies have already publicly rejected having anything to do with tobacco sponsorship but without a much stronger lead from central government it is very hard to see how young girls and young women are going to escape continued heavy targeting by tobacco companies determined to find new young smokers to replace those older smokers either giving up or dying from smoking related diseases.

Reducing the number of young girls who take up smoking is only half of the government's new commitment to reducing smoking among women. Adult women also need to be helped to give up their addiction to cigarettes. The main emphasis in *The Health of the Nation* is on health education and support programmes for individual women who must ultimately choose for themselves whether or not to continue with such health damaging behaviour. Well before the Green and White Papers were published, however, the government must have been aware of research already published which strongly suggested that women's smoking behaviour was determined to a significant extent by factors which would be quite unaltered by the type of individualistic approach to the problem adopted by the Department of Health. Qualitative research by Hilary Graham has demonstrated that for women living with children in poverty cigarette smoking is regarded as a necessity rather than a luxury. Women looking after small children on very low incomes have stated that smoking is the one thing that they do for themselves, that it keeps them calm in extremely stressful circumstances and stops them taking things out on their children. In Graham's survey of 57 women caring for preschool children in low income families, nearly half noted that they lost their temper easily and all these women identified smoking 'as a major coping strategy when they felt they could no longer handle the demands of their children' (Graham 1987: 54). One woman commented,

> I think smoking stops me getting so irritable. I can cope with things better. If I was economising, I'd cut down on cigarettes but I wouldn't give up. I'd stop eating ... food just isn't that important to me but having a cigarette is the only thing I do just for myself.
>
> (Graham 1987: 55)

Research findings such as this strongly indicate that the last thing most female smokers need is yet more health information about the damage they are doing to their own health and the health of their children. As ASH's 1993 report on women and smoking and low income concluded, 'It is not possible to be concerned about women's smoking without being concerned about women. In this context the campaigns of the anti-poverty lobby are integral to a tobacco control strategy' (ASH, Working Group on Women and Smoking 1993: 33).

Women and alcohol

Women are drinking more alcohol today than they used to, and whilst there is some evidence to suggest that men's overall consumption of alcohol actually fell during the 1980s, women's consumption, although still much lower than men's, continued to rise (Secretary of State for Health 1991: 108). This trend, with a concomitant rise in 'problem' drinking amongst women, has given rise to warning headlines such as 'Drink peril faces women keeping up with the boys' (*The Guardian*, 3 December 1991). The rise in problem drinking amongst women has even been described as 'the ransom of emancipation'. There is certainly some statistical evidence of an increase in alcohol related harm in women. For example, between 1979 and 1984 female deaths from chronic liver disease and cirrhosis rose by 9 per cent and female admissions to mental hospitals for alcohol misuse rose 60 per cent between 1977 and 1986 (Alcohol Concern 1988). Worried women should note, however, that these rises were based on a very small baseline and cirrhosis of the liver is still not a major cause of female deaths in England and Wales. In 1987, for example, there were only 412 female adult deaths from alcohol related liver disease (Duffy 1992: 37). Emphasizing percentage increases without also indicating baseline figures is just one way in which the anti-alcohol lobby may exaggerate the risks faced by women who drink.

Given the alarmist tone of much health promotion material on alcohol, what is truly remarkable is the lack of good statistical evidence on women's drinking habits and in particular the effects of such drinking on their health and well-being. August medical bodies such as the Royal College of Physicians and the Royal College of Psychiatrists now agree that women may well put their health at risk if they drink more than 14 units of alcohol a week (one unit being a pub measure of gin or – very approximately – one glass of wine). When I asked a small unrepresentative sample of female friends and acquaintances what they thought might happen to them if they regularly drank more than 14 units of alcohol per week, all of them spontaneously 'guessed' that they would risk damaging their livers. Yet when I researched the medical literature for proof of this widely assumed risk of relatively moderate female drinking, I found that women did not appear to be being given the whole truth by health promoters and educationists. According to the Royal College of Physicians

(1987) the 'fact' that women's safe level of drinking is less than 14 units per week has 'been agreed by all bodies active in the field'. This may well be true, but unless such an agreement has been based on clear, sound empirical evidence of harm which results from women drinking above that limit such a statement is seriously misleading. Even more specific claims of harm turn out, on fuller investigation, to be based on very thin evidence. For example, the Royal College of Psychiatrists claimed in *Alcohol: Our Favourite Drug* that while the development of cirrhosis in women is 'usually' associated with daily intakes of four units a day (i.e. 28 units a week) intakes of approximately two standard drinks a day in women 'have been linked with a significant increase in the risk of developing cirrhosis' (Royal College of Psychiatrists 1986: 93). They did not however give any references to any research studies which could back up such a claim. Similarly, the government's *The Health of The Nation and You* stated that 'medical advice is that if women drink more than 14 units of alcohol a week on a regular basis they increase the risk of damaging their health' but give no actual evidence to back up this advice (Department of Health 1992). An editorial in the *British Journal of Addiction* (1988) which claimed that 'women with cirrhosis drink on average less alcohol than men. Consumption may be as low as 2–5 units daily' (Dunne 1988: 1135) did at least give a reference to a study which presumably supported this claim. This study, however, turned out to be a very small scale study of 37 Australian women with a first diagnosis of cirrhosis of the liver. What the researchers in this study actually concluded was that 90 per cent of the women identified as having cirrhosis of the liver admitted to drinking more than five units of alcohol daily (i.e. more than 35 units a week). The researchers found only *one* woman with cirrhosis who insisted that she drank only 30 grams daily and concluded 'the absolute risk of developing alcohol related cirrhosis at levels of consumption between 3 to 5 units daily is undoubtedly slight' (Norton *et al.* 1987: 82).

According to John Duffy, a senior lecturer in statistics and researcher into alcohol related disease, the ideal data source for the purpose of determining the exact relationship between alcohol consumption and liver disease would be a large follow-up study of a random sample of the population of England and Wales with full information on their drinking habits until some of them developed cirrhosis of the liver. However, given that the death rate from this disease is so low, Duffy concedes that such a huge sample would be needed as to render such a study totally uneconomic. Duffy has collated all the epidemiological evidence which is available on this disease. Significantly only one major study of morbidity (Pequignot 1974) included any data on women. Mortality studies provided so little data on women that Duffy did not even attempt to calculate the risk of death from cirrhosis of the liver for women who drink (Duffy 1992: 38). In other words, the data simply does not exist to allow medical experts to give even rough guesstimates of women's risk of getting this particular disease at different levels of alcohol consumption. But perhaps the medical experts have other health risks in mind when they warn women against drinking more than 14 units of alcohol per week?

Whilst women themselves may assume that the main health risk from 'heavy' drinking is cirrhosis of the liver, medical experts have also expressed serious concern over apparent links between alcohol consumption and breast cancer. Duffy and Sharples have reviewed 29 studies of alcohol and female breast cancer and found that 12 out of 19 retrospective case-control studies found a significant or almost significant predisposing effect of alcohol consumption. Duffy and Sharples discuss a number of weaknesses in many of these studies but conclude nevertheless, 'It is reasonable to infer that alcohol and breast cancer risk are related' (1992: 102) and that

> While there is no consensus on a causal relationship, until the effect of alcohol consumption can be convincingly accounted for by adjustment for other variables, it must be treated as a predisposing factor.
>
> (Duffy and Sharples 1992: 105)

Unfortunately for health promotion campaigns and women drinkers, Duffy and Sharples also concluded that the studies they reviewed suggested that the risk of breast cancer was most significantly related to any drinking at all compared to being teetotal. In order to save significant numbers of women's lives per year women would have to stop drinking altogether, hardly a realistic public health goal. Achieving just a moderate decline in women's average alcohol consumption would apparently only be likely to reduce the risk of breast cancer by about 1 per cent. If this prediction is accurate it suggests that the current advice to women to limit their drinking to a safe 14 units a week is neither here nor there as far as the possibility of reducing the risk of breast cancer is concerned.

Some drinkers, including women, have recently begun to console themselves with the knowledge that epidemiological research has now suggested that drinkers are less likely than non-drinkers to suffer from cardiovascular disease. Cohen and Duffy for example conclude from the review of research studies in this area that 'alcohol consumed at moderate levels does indeed have a protective effect' (Cohen and Duffy 1992: 46). Before women rejoice too soon, however, they should take note that yet again there is too little research data on women, alcohol and cardiovascular disease for Cohen and Duffy even to give the issue their consideration.

If good data on the precise risks to women of drinking alcohol 'lightly', 'moderately' or 'heavily' is so scarce why has the health promotion industry united in attempting to persuade all women to restrict their drinking to less than 14 units a week? One theory popular amongst the anti-alcohol lobby is that a significant reduction in overall alcohol related harm in society is much more likely to be achieved by a reduction in overall/average consumption than by programmes targeted on heavy or problem drinkers. For example, according to Peter Anderson in the *British Medical Journal*'s answer to *The Health of the Nation,*

> The mean alcohol consumption of a community and the prevalence of heavy drinking are highly correlated ($r = 0.97$), such that a mean reduction of alcohol consumption of 10% would correspond with a fall of about 10% in the number of heavy drinkers.
>
> (Anderson 1991: 124)

Anderson therefore suggests that a population strategy aimed at getting everyone to reduce their alcohol consumption has greater potential for reducing overall alcohol related harm and for encouraging heavy drinkers to drink less. Unusually for those concerned with health education Anderson openly admits that such prevention measures which could clearly bring much benefit to the population as a whole 'offer little to each participating individual' (Anderson 1991: 125). Given that much of the social harm caused by excessive alcohol consumption, such as deaths and injuries from drunken driving and alcohol related assaults, is primarily caused by *male* drinkers (see McConville 1983: 63), a cynical woman might conclude that the health promotion industry is advising her to cut her alcohol consumption primarily for the good of society as a whole rather than her own physical and emotional well-being. However, even if women were prepared to accept the quite convincing arguments in favour of an overall reduction in alcohol consumption, they might well still question the key method currently being used to achieve such a reduction.

One of the simplest ways to cut overall alcohol consumption in any society is to raise its relative cost. In 1981–82, for example, overall consumption of alcohol fell by 11 per cent in Britain due to the combined effect of the recession on consumer spending and an increase in excise duty on beer and spirits in the 1981 budget (Anderson 1991: 125). In contrast education campaigns are known to be very ineffective in terms of altering drinking behaviour. According to the Royal College of Psychiatrists, for example, health education campaigns 'can often be shown to have made their target audience better informed and even to have altered their attitudes but they have not yet been shown to alter actual drinking behaviour' (1986: 115). In other words the anti-alcohol lobby and the health promotion industry may well succeed in educating women to feel guilty and worried about their alcohol consumption but their drinking behaviour will continue to be more influenced by the ready availability and relative low cost of alcohol. So why does the government not take the simplest and most effective prevention measure and significantly increase excise duty on all alcoholic drinks? The answer is already well known, and well rehearsed. The government has a very large vested interest in a thriving drinks industry which not only provides the Treasury with £4 billion plus revenue each year but also provides jobs, export earnings and even Conservative Party election funds. All this is common knowledge; what is perhaps less well understood is that the anti-alcohol lobby has vested interests too – albeit on a much smaller scale – which may lead it to exaggerate the health risks of alcohol consumption. According to Jancis Robinson

The anti-alcohol campaigners have been almost goaded into sensationalism by the fact that whilst the government spent nearly £1m per user death in 1986 combatting illegal drugs and solvent use the comparable figure for alcohol abuse was £100.

'No wonder', she comments, 'those whose job it is to study, on slivers of budgets, the drinking problems of the nation feel entitled to make a fuss' (Robinson, 1988: 7).

If the scientific evidence that drinking more than 14 units of alcohol a week poses a significant threat to women's health is noticeable by its absence, what about the evidence that drinking during pregnancy is harmful to the unborn child? In 1977 a British medical expert concluded, 'From the public health point of view the evidence at the moment is not strong enough to justify any statement that women who drink moderately during pregnancy are harming their unborn child' (Kessel cited by Plant 1987: 16). By 1983, however, the Health Education Council claimed

More and more doctors think it is wise to avoid alcohol during pregnancy. So if you are pregnant or planning a pregnancy NEVER drink heavily or frequently and certainly avoid binges. Best of all stay off alcohol altogether until your baby is born.

(in Plant 1987: 16)

'Best of all' for 'baby' presumably since a woman undergoing the stresses and strains of pregnancy might well enjoy the occasional alcoholic drink or even need a drink as a mild anti-stress device. On what sound scientific evidence are 'more and more' doctors now recommending complete or virtual abstinence from alcohol throughout pregnancy and even during conception?

According to the popular press, particularly the American press, medical evidence of the dangers of even light drinking during pregnancy is now clear cut. The *New York Times*, for example, claimed that 'as little as one drink during pregnancy can lead to intellectual and physical defects in the baby' (cited by Stellman and Bertin 1990: A23) As is so often the case, however, when the medical research reports themselves are carefully scrutinized no such dramatic conclusions can be reached. One of the key problems with research into alcohol consumption during pregnancy is that many studies fail to define clearly terms such as 'light' and 'moderate' drinking. Some studies have defined heavy drinking as 'averaging 2 or more drinks a day' or even 'one or more'. As Genevieve Knupfer has pointed out

Such methodological errors make it impossible to ascertain whether whatever fetal damage is found comes from cases of mothers who drank 2 drinks a day or from mothers who drank 20 drinks a day. Thus when we

see headlines such as 'One drink a day affects baby's IQ' we should be sure
to remember the strong possibility that what the research actually showed
was the affect of 'one or more drinks a day'.

(1991: 1072)

Knupfer concluded her review of the weaknesses of current research into
alcohol consumption as a causal factor in fetal harm by remarking that
common sense should lead us to conclude that light drinking during pregnancy
would be very unlikely to cause fetal damage and suggesting that the strong
popular anti-alcohol tide in relation to pregnant women might well be
influenced by 'prejudice against women drinking' (Knupfer 1991). Significantly Knupfer's claims drew the response from other experts in the field that
because there is no definite proof that light intake of alcohol is harmless to the
unborn child it would only be 'responsible to advise women to avoid drinking
during pregnancy' (Day 1991: 1058). This approach does have some merit but
the message that medical experts simply lack definitive knowledge which
would show light drinking during pregnancy to be completely harmless is
hardly the message implied in statements such as 'many doctors now advise
women to avoid alcohol altogether during pregnancy'. Pregnant women may
well assume that this means doctors now have good evidence that light
drinking is harmful rather than that they simply cannot state categorically that
it is harmless. Studies which do suggest that light drinking during pregnancy is
unlikely to be harmful certainly have not received as much media hype as
studies purporting to show the opposite. For example, how many women are
aware of Plant's findings that even drinking over four units of alcohol on
maximum drinking days did not emerge as a substantial predictor of fetal
harm? The main predictors of fetal harm in her study were tobacco and illegal
drug use which were related to 'heavy' drinking so that the apparent
association between drinking and fetal harm was not causal. Plant concluded
that, 'At the present time and with available knowledge statements about
moderate drinking in pregnancy should not be alarmist' (Plant 1987: 103). In
1991 a study measuring infants' mental and motor development at 18 months
of age actually found that 'After confounding factors had been controlled for,
alcohol consumption before pregnancy and after pregnancy was significantly
related to better motor performance and mental performance' (Forrest et al.
1991: 22) The researchers suggested that pregnant women could safely drink
up to eight units of alcohol a week – the equivalent of about one drink a day
(Forrest et al. 1991). Unfortunately these optimistic messages do not appear to
be getting through to either the health promotion industry or to pregnant
women themselves. Understandably the anti-alcohol lobby is not at all
interested in publicizing such reassuring findings and the medical profession
appears unwilling to allow pregnant women to make up their own minds
about drinking in pregnancy on the basis of full information on both reassuring
and less reassuring research studies.

Whilst medical experts cannot yet agree amongst themselves on the risks – or lack of them – of light to moderate drinking by pregnant women, all medical experts in this field are agreed that very heavy drinking by alcoholic women during pregnancy can cause fetal alcohol syndrome (FAS) which leads to long term mental disabilities and behaviour problems in a small number of children. Since the term fetal alcohol syndrome was first used in 1973 in an article in *The Lancet*, the medical profession has shown an ever-growing interest in this problem (Ettorre 1992). Feminist health commentators, however, have recently exposed the way in which the existence of this syndrome is being used to exert increased control over all pregnant women. Elizabeth Ettorre, for example, sees medical concern over FAS as part of a wider move towards seeing the fetus as a patient in its own right and suggests that the issues of FAS and fetal rights more generally must both be linked to 'the vested interests of the medical profession in keeping pregnant women under increasing surveillance and control' (Ettorre 1992: 49).

American feminists have also pointed out that calls for alcoholic pregnant women to be prosecuted for harming the fetus and/or imprisoned during pregnancy as a preventive health measure totally ignore the social and environmental factors which push some poor women into illegal drug and alcohol abuse. The direct impact of poverty on pregnant women's health and the serious birth defects which can be caused by industrial pollutants receive far less attention from the medical profession and the popular press than women's behaviour. According to Katha Pollitt (1990) if women cannot be blamed for a child's ill health then apparently no one is to blame. Men's behaviour also escapes the concern and punitive controls now being advocated for 'deviant' pregnant women. Many pregnant women suffer violent attacks from their male partners. Where is the research into the effects of such attacks on fetal health and development? Where are the demands for violent men to change *their* behaviour in order to protect the health of *their* unborn children? (Pollitt 1990).

Women and diet

Women living in late twentieth century western capitalist countries appear to have an increasingly problematic relationship with food. According to *Options* magazine (January 1993) 50 per cent of British women suffer from disordered eating. Ninety per cent of women think they weigh too much, while only 21 per cent are medically overweight. Sixty-six per cent of British women diet sporadically while 15 per cent are on permanent diets. Britain has 3.5 million anorexics and bulimics, 95 per cent of them female. Whilst fighting their own usually losing battle with food, women as wives and mothers are still held primarily responsible for feeding their families. Most women still spend significant amounts of their time planning meals, shopping for food, preparing and cooking meals and snacks and then clearing away the debris before beginning the whole process all over again. A few 'new' men may now regularly 'help' with food shopping, cooking and washing up but very few husbands and fathers take primary responsibility for meeting their family's nutritional requirements.

The food industry bombards women consumers with very sophisticated advertising designed to increase the sales of particular food products and dishes. In particular the food industry has recently latched on to the concept of a 'healthy' diet and increasingly advertises so called 'healthy' foods which will 'protect' husbands and children from a range of nutritionally linked diseases and problems. Mothers must now ensure not only that their families have enough to eat but that they eat the right sorts of foods in order to lead long and healthy lives. We all know, for example, that Flora margarine produces a 'blooming generation' and is good for the heart, despite the fact – little known by many confused consumers – that it contains just as much fat and as many calories as butter, albeit fat of a supposedly 'healthier' kind. Certain breakfast cereals and whole ranges of ready made dishes have also been marketed as 'good' for us.

Some women may be wary of the wide range of dubious health advice dished out to them by essentially money making food and diet companies (the Weight Watchers brand is of course a subsidiary of Heinz) but they are usually far less aware of the extent to which the dietary advice given to them by the public sector health promotion industry is almost equally open to serious question. Women are now being specifically targeted by health promotion workers as key figures in their design to push the whole nation towards 'healthier' eating. Officially a 'healthy' diet is now one which is lower in saturated fats and higher in high fibre foods such as grains, fruits and vegetables than the one currently consumed by Britain's average family. This 'healthy' diet must also be low in salt and sugar. According to the Department of Health's *The Health of the Nation and You* booklet,

> Eating healthily does not mean that we have to give up all the things we like. It means . . . eating more fibre rich starchy foods like bread, pasta, rice and potatoes and going easy on fatty, sugary and salty foods
> (Department of Health 1992)

The booklet gives 'Tips about Healthy Eating' which include 'Grill food instead of frying it' and 'Eat fish, poultry or the leaner cuts of meat. Go easy on cakes and biscuits – try fruit instead . . . Eat plenty of vegetables and salads'. This booklet was the populist version of *The Health of the Nation* which based its proposals on advice from the Committee on Medical Aspects of Food Policy (COMA). The Green Paper set specific targets for the year 2000 which included

> the proportion of the population who derive less than 15% of their food energy from saturated fatty acids should be at least 60% [currently 85% of people consume more saturated fats than this] and the proportion of the

population who derive less than 35% of their total food intake from fat should be at least 50%.

(Secretary of State for Health 1991: 70)

It also claimed that 'It is clear that many people could improve their dietary habits, thereby reducing the burden of diet-related ill-health' (Secretary of State for Health 1991: 69). One of the two principal means the government put forward to achieve these dietary targets was 'education, advice and information about the need for balanced diets as part of a healthy lifestyle' (Secretary of State for Health 1991: 69).

Local branches of the health promotion industry have been quick to begin to implement this strategy. Their messages about healthier eating are being picked up and magnified by the popular press. For example according to the *Manchester Evening News* (3 November 1992)

> The hand that rocks the cradle could be held to blame for the death of a nation or hold the key to health. Women have traditionally been taught the way to a man's heart is through his stomach. Now women are being taken to task for feeding families the killer fats believed to contribute to heart disease . . . Researchers have concluded that pot bellied businessmen with sweated brows are the by-product of a poorly planned shopping list. Because wives and mothers still do most of the shopping it is they who determine the family's diet and it is therefore their fault.

Dr Jo Wallsworth-Bell, northwest regional consultant in primary health care agreed that women daily make the life or death decisions for their loved ones. She believed that by targeting women with health education information in the way advertising agencies do, women could help save lives and the £500 million a year spent on treating heart trouble.

This popular journalistic piece neatly contains all the fallacies currently promoted by the health promotion industry. First, it assumes that women buying food for their families have a relatively free choice over that food consumption. Second, it assumes that a diet high in saturated fat is a key cause of heart disease. Third, it assumes that if women can be persuaded to feed their families a 'healthier', i.e. less fatty diet, the incidence of heart disease will decline significantly. We will now examine each of these assumptions in turn.

The current Conservative government and its closely related predecessors are particularly strongly wedded to the doctrine of individual free choice and responsibility. Government health ministers have argued that if the working classes eat less healthy diets than their middle and upper-class counterparts this is primarily due to habits and lack of education rather than poverty or material deprivation. Edwina Currie publicly espoused this view in 1986 when she claimed that northerners were dying of ignorance rather than poverty (Currie 1989: 17).

Recent empirical evidence does show a clear class gap in relation to health related behaviours. For example, the Household Food Consumption and

Expenditure surveys found that 43 per cent of all women in professional families claimed to use low fat or polyunsaturated spreads compared to only 15 per cent of women in unskilled families (Cox *et al.* 1987). Blaxter's health and lifestyles survey found that eating a 'good' diet was strongly correlated to education and that this correlation was stronger than the one between income and diet except for women aged 40–59 (Blaxter 1990). Her findings give some support to Edwina Currie's controversial emphasis on ignorance rather than poverty as the key cause of unhealthy eating habits. On the other hand a number of studies of the very poorest families in Britain, those living long term on state benefits or living in homeless families' accommodation, have persistently found that mothers in such families simply cannot afford to feed them the current version of a healthy diet. Hilary Graham's small scale survey of households living on incomes at or below Supplementary Benefit (now Income Support) level found that mothers in such families cut down on expenditure on food whenever money was needed for more fixed items of expenditure such as rent.

> Food's the only place I find I can tighten up. The rest of it they take before you get your hands on it really. So it's the food ... The only thing I can cut down is food ... You've got to balance nutrition with a large amount of food that will keep them not hungry. I'd like to give them fresh fruit whereas the good food has to be limited.
>
> (Graham 1993: 155)

Women in poor families and indeed in non-poor families are also constrained in their choice of food by the declared likes and dislikes of their husbands and children. For example Charles and Kerr found in their study of York households that because men preferred chips and grills to salads their wives tended to cook these rather than their own preferred foods (Charles and Kerr 1986). As Hilary Graham has pointed out, given the evidence that arguments about food and food preparation are sometimes the trigger for husbands' violence against their wives women can hardly be held responsible for giving in to their partners' 'less healthy' food preferences (Graham 1993).

If mothers in very poor families cannot afford to feed them what they 'know' to be healthy diets, mothers of homeless families often face even greater hurdles to providing themselves and their children with a 'good' diet. A survey of homeless families undertaken in the late 1980s found that 20 out of the 48 women surveyed were eating a 'poor' diet: 'There was a heavy reliance on take-aways, cakes and snacks and on pre-packaged convenience foods' (Conway 1988: 58). Some health visitors interviewed in the same survey felt that the children's diet in such families 'almost amounts to malnutrition standards in some cases' (Conway 1988: 72).

One group of women in particular who constantly receive official advice about the importance of a good diet are pregnant women; such advice is usually an integral part of antenatal care and most pregnant women will receive some literature advising them on 'healthy' eating during pregnancy. But whilst health educators have fully acknowledged the importance of a 'good' diet during pregnancy very little official or medical attention has been paid to whether or not all pregnant women can afford to eat well during their pregnancy. In 1988 the Maternity Alliance published the results of a study designed to estimate the cost of diets currently recommended by hospital antenatal clinics and to relate this cost to the income levels of expectant mothers. The study concluded that 'the cost of an adequate diet for an expectant mother may be beyond the means of families on benefits or on low wages' (Durward 1988: 14). In particular it suggested that young single women would be 'particularly hard pressed' to eat well. After buying a 'good' diet a 16 or 17-year-old living with parents or friends would be left with only £4.10 a week to pay for transport, clothes and all other household and personal costs. The study concluded

> providing adequate resources for women in poverty is the only means of enabling them to do all they can to ensure the good health of their future babies. A society which values the health and welfare of its children can do no less.
>
> (Durward 1988: 15)

So far we have shown that far from dying of ignorance by wilfully choosing to eat unhealthily, many poor women are forced to feed themselves and their families what they believe to be unhealthy diets primarily because 'healthy' foods are more expensive, less easily obtained and prepared and less popular with their husbands and children. These women are probably completely unaware that well away from the public gaze the 'experts' are now seriously disputing the relationship between a low fat, low salt, high fibre diet and a reduction in the major killer diseases of our time. Recent research findings, widely reported within the medical journals but not yet picked up and widely publicized by either politicians or the media, strongly suggest that the 'relatively painless' dietary changes now being officially advocated are highly unlikely to have any significant effect on the incidence of heart disease or cancer. There are two key reasons for such a pessimistic view of health prevention through dietary change. First, the type of dietary changes achieved by educating a free living group of subjects have proved to be relatively small. Second, the evidence that if achieved major dietary changes would save lives is also now seriously challenged. Let us examine each of these claims more fully in turn.

An article in the *British Medical Journal* by Ramsay *et al.* (1991) studied the results of 16 trials which had used diet to lower serum cholesterol concentrations, mainly in men. The authors concluded that the type of dietary change now being advocated by the government, the so-called Step 1 diet, has 'a meagre effect on cholesterol concentration in free living subjects' (Ramsay *et al.* 1991: 955). Much more rigorous diets had been shown to reduce cholesterol concentrations 'substantially' but such diets were 'unpalatable' and involved massive changes to subjects' eating habits. The authors concluded, 'It seems that the dietary treatment must be unpleasant to be effective' (Ramsay *et al.* 1991: 956) – just the opposite of the official message on a healthy diet currently being thrust down everyone's throats, that the changes we all need to make do 'not mean that we have to give up all the things we like' (Department of Health 1992). The authors of this article concluded that whilst relatively minor dietary changes such as a small reduction in the proportion of fat in the nation's diet may be 'harmless' in themselves, the promotion of such dietary changes may be considered harmful in the sense that scarce resources are being wasted on useless intervention programmes.

Whilst Ramsey *et al.* strongly criticized the assumption that relatively painless dietary changes can significantly affect cholesterol levels in an at-risk population they did not challenge the more fundamental assumption that lowering cholesterol levels in any given population would significantly reduce the incidence of heart disease within that population and thus save many lives lost prematurely. Yet other research findings now being presented in the medical journals are beginning to shoot some very large holes into this theory. For example in 1992 an editorial in the *British Medical Journal* entitled 'Doubts about preventing coronary heart disease' cited the results of a major Swedish trial which did reduce serum cholesterol levels in more than 10,000 middle aged men over a 10 year period and yet the rate of deaths from coronary heart disease was unchanged (Oliver 1992: 393).

Finally and crucially as far as women are concerned, it is essential to realize that virtually all of the research into the link between high blood cholesterol levels and heart disease has been carried out exclusively on middle aged men. Yet the health promotion industry insists that women as well as men need to cut down the levels of saturated fats in their diet. However an editorial in *Circulation* in September 1992 pointed out that one of the very few studies in this area which included women as research subjects found that 'among women high blood cholesterol is not associated with all-cause mortality nor even with cardiovascular mortality' (Hulley *et al.* 1992: 1027) In other words this very large scale study found that high blood cholesterol levels in women did *not* increase their risk of dying from some form of cardiovascular disease. This most surprising finding appears to be explained by the fact that low blood cholesterol levels actually increase women's risk of dying from a stroke. Middle aged women are more at risk of dying from a stroke than middle aged men and far less at risk of dying from a heart attack which is associated with high blood cholesterol levels. The editorial concluded – somewhat phlegmatically given advice to women on cholesterol – that this key sex difference

> calls into question the general practice of extrapolating to women the findings from epidemiological studies and clinical trials in men. With the exception of those who already have coronary disease or other reasons for

being at a comparable very high risk of CHD [coronary hear disease] death it no longer seems wise to screen for and treat high blood cholesterol in women.

(Hulley *et al.* 1992: 1028)

This remarkable statement must surely make all women extremely wary of accepting any health promotion advice on changing their diets. Not only does it appear that reducing the proportion of dairy fats in their diet may well not protect women from cardiovascular disease, it may also actually increase women's risk of suffering from the effects of osteoporosis in later life. In a misguided attempt to protect themselves from one disease women may cut right back on their consumption of dairy products such as cheese and thus dangerously reduce their intake of calcium which is so important in protecting their bone density.

If eating a less fatty diet protects neither men nor women from premature death from cardiovascular disease why are women still being told by virtually all health experts that they should reduce their own and their families' consumption of saturated fats? According to James Le Fanu, the many protagonists of the diet/disease thesis have been more or less deliberately misleading governments, the medical profession and, of course, the general public since at least the mid-1980s (Le Fanu 1987). Le Fanu argues that for many the motivation for such deception remains opaque, but it is clear that there is much money to be made from the anti-cholesterol industry. In 1985, for example, worried Americans spent an estimated $100 million on measuring their cholesterol levels (Le Fanu 1987: 154). In Britain cholesterol measuring has yet to reach such heights but in the early 1990s Boots, for example, began to advertise a 'do-it-yourself' cholesterol testing kit which even some protagonists of the cholesterol causes heart disease theory dismissed as a worse than useless gadget. Whilst it is fairly obvious that drugs companies and test kit manufacturers hope to make large profits from the anti-cholesterol bandwagon, it is less obvious, but nevertheless important to note, that many individuals are now employed by the public sector within the health education field and that promoting a 'healthy' diet makes up a significant part of their workload. Moreover both the government and many renowned epidemiologists, scientists and health educationists would clearly have saturated fatty egg all over their faces if they had to admit that their advice on eggs and other high cholesterol food stuffs was worse than useless. In case readers are outraged at such an heretical comment, it is worth remembering that only 50 years ago the expert view on nutrition was that the working class's diet was responsible for a great deal of ill health. It was deficient in all those foods essential to growth and good health, such as full cream milk, dairy products, eggs and red meat (see Le Fanu 1987).

Whilst heart disease is still the leading cause of death in both sexes, for women between the ages of 35 and 53 breast cancer is the commonest cause of death, and is far more common than heart disease which is primarily a disease of post-menopausal women. Just as health educationists have emphasized the apparent links between diet and heart disease, so also have they attempted to make links between individuals' diets and their risk of cancer. In the 1980s the dominant epidemiological hypothesis was that differences in the consumption of animal fats was the primary cause of the large differences in rates of breast cancer between countries. On the basis of this hypothesis western women have been advised by the 'experts' to reduce the amount of fat in their diets. For example, according to Carolyn Faulder's *The Women's Cancer Book*,

> 35% [of cancers] are [now] attributed to diet ... But there are positive things we can do for ourselves ... In this country we eat 20% more saturated fat than we should ... the Prudent Diet ... really is not that difficult ... It means cutting down on your consumption of red meat, dairy products, sugar ...
>
> (Faulder 1989: 181)

According to a review article by Willett in *Nature*, however, the evidence simply does not support the hypothesis that high fat consumption is a causal factor in breast cancer and

> In adult women a modest reduction in dietary fat and avoiding obesity seems likely to have little, if any, impact on reducing the risk of breast cancer. On the contrary accumulating data indicate that being thin before the menopause may actually increase the risk of breast cancer.
>
> (Willett 1989: 393)

According to Baruch Modan theories linking diet to different types of cancer are 'still in the twilight zone' yet already dietary prevention has become a multimillion dollar industry (Modan 1992). Modan points out that the currently 'healthy' diet is not without risk and that even the totally virtuous green vegetable may be high in pesticides whilst goody, goody fishes may be loaded with mercury. She concludes that environmental risk factors such as chemical pollutants are probably much more strongly related to cancer than individuals' diet choices but that

> combating these carcinogenic substances is far less simple than advocating change of diet. It would mean either compromising the luxuries of the 21st century or an uphill battle against industry ... In contrast adoption of certain dietary measures presents little burden. The data may be marginal but the economic harvest is wild, new products can be developed such as no-meat hamburgers ... salt-free pretzels and just around the corner non-fatty fat that looks like fat, tastes like fat and will doubtless cost much more than fat. The promotion of these new products not only diverts

attention from certain real causes of cancer but also stimulates the economy and gives the public a false sense of security.

(Modan 1992: 163)

Discussion

The health promotion industry may not be as profitable or prestigious as high technology 'curative' health care but it is a growing industry which employs large numbers of workers on relatively high salaries. Many of these workers are absolutely convinced that their health promotion activities will eventually improve the health of the nation. However, our analysis of health promotion strategies in relation to women's smoking, drinking and dietary habits suggests that they may be far less beneficial than virtually everyone in our society now believes. This pessimistic conclusion is based on three key themes which can be drawn out of our analysis. First, the official health advice being given to women is not always based on strong scientific evidence. Indeed the information given to women about their diet, its effects on their blood cholesterol level and the effect of that level on their risk of serious disease now appears to be almost completely erroneous. Second, health promotion strategies aimed specifically at women have sometimes been clearly designed to control women's behaviour for the benefit of others, particularly their unborn children. Many doctors and policy makers appear to regard women primarily as reproducers or even baby carriers, whose irresponsible behaviour threatens the health and well-being of the fetus. For example, an editorial in *The New England Journal of Medicine* in 1987 having noted the known dangers of lung cancer and excess coronary heart disease amongst women smokers continued,

> Perhaps the worst consequences of smoking by women are the effects on reproduction and on children ... Most troubling is the growing body of evidence *suggesting* that maternal smoking during pregnancy has long term effects on children.
>
> (Fielding 1987: 1344; my emphasis)

The editorial openly admitted that evidence which links smoking in pregnancy to, for example, deficits in children's intellectual development was far from conclusive. It nevertheless went on to advocate

> an urgent need for aggressive efforts on the part of physicians (and other health care workers) ... to inform women fully about the risks associated with smoking. At a minimum pregnant women must understand that giving their unborn child the best chance of being normal at birth and of surviving the perinatal period requires that they stop smoking.
>
> (Fielding 1987: 1344)

In the United States a powerful lobby has begun to demand not only that pregnant women totally abstain from any behaviours that might harm the fetus but that women who continue to take drugs or drink heavily during pregnancy should be imprisoned. In Wyoming a pregnant woman was arrested for drinking after going to hospital for treatment of injuries inflicted by her husband. The charge against her was later dropped but no charges were ever instituted against her husband for assault (Pollitt 1990). In Britain concern over pregnant women's behaviour has not yet reached such punitive levels but there is a clear trend towards demanding that women conform to ever more stringent guidelines on healthy behaviour during pregnancy.

The third and final theme which emerges from a critical analysis of current health promotion strategies is the extent to which they individualize women's health problems and the solutions to them. Women are now strongly advised that it is up to them to take responsibility not only for their own health but also for the health of their families. Yet socio/medical research studies into women's health related behaviours have strongly demonstrated the extent to which these behaviours are very powerfully influenced by socioeconomic factors.

Whilst central government has continued to emphasize individual choice and responsibility as opposed to the structural causes of inequalities in health and so-called healthy behaviours, contemporary health promotion theory fully acknowledges the links between structural factors such as poverty and gender injustices and women's 'unhealthy' behaviours. Many local health authorities have now begun to accept the advice of researchers that

> Health promotion must be integrally linked with strategic policies developed by local government and health authorities in order to present a combined approach to tackling the health and social needs of women in the poorest areas of the community.
>
> (Wells and Batten 1990: 60)

Many health promotion workers have attempted to design local health promotion projects which fully acknowledge the key role which material deprivation and concomitant powerlessness play in the lives of the poorest sections of our community. For example in 1990 local health authorities in Birmingham joined forces with the city council to offer local people a partnership in promoting health by directly tackling the issue of inner city deprivation (Moore 1992). At first local people appeared apathetic but once they did begin to participate in the project they complained vociferously that having defined their own health needs the various local authorities took no notice of them. Some health workers also expressed anger and disillusionment at the gap between the idealism of the aim of the project and its total failure to prevent worsening poverty, unemployment and appalling housing conditions in the inner city area. One health visitor involved in the project graphically summed up the difficulties of health promotion exercises in the midst of extreme deprivation:

> When she visits families where children suffer bronchial complaints because of damp housing, their mother has slashed her face out of sheer

frustration and her husband is out of work, she feels disinclined to suggest the parents should give up smoking for the health of their children.

(Moore 1992: 10)

On the ground experiences such as the one outlined above raise the centrally important question of whether even health promotion projects with built-in 'structural awareness' will not prove to be inherently ineffective. The radical rhetoric of many local health promotion projects tends to disguise the central fact that resources for health promotion are still primarily resources for health workers and state bureaucrats rather than resources for those with the health needs. Given the mass of data now linking unhealthy behaviours amongst women to poverty and women's caring burdens, it might make much more sense to bypass the health service completely and use any resources saved to provide women themselves with the type of practical and financial support which they require to overcome the powerful social and economic disadvantages which both directly injure their health and indirectly push them into relatively unhealthy behaviours.

8

WOMEN, HIV AND AIDS

Despite the relatively recent discovery of the virus which 'causes' AIDS or acquired immune deficiency syndrome in 1984 and despite the initial assumption that AIDS was a 'gay plague', a remarkably large body of literature has now been produced on women, the human immunodeficiency virus (HIV) and AIDS. Numerous populist books and pamphlets can now be bought by women seeking 'the truth' about AIDS. Since AIDS is almost universally perceived to be a fatal and primarily sexually transmitted disease, women's fears and concerns about HIV/AIDS are entirely understandable. Unfortunately women seeking information about their own risk of developing AIDS will find that virtually all of the advice now available to them has been produced by a burgeoning AIDS industry which has a vested interest – if not a whole range of vested interests – in promoting the view that AIDS is now, or will be in the very near future, a major lethal threat to all women who are in any way sexually active. Women who pick up virtually any health promotion literature on HIV/AIDS will learn 'scientific facts' about AIDS intended to frighten them into changing their individual sexual behaviour before it is too late. They will also learn that women, or indeed men, cannot be divided into high risk and low risk groups in relation to HIV/AIDS. It is simply risky behaviour which spreads this disease, it is what one does, not who one is which counts. If on the other hand women restrict their education about HIV/AIDS to reading about them in the popular press, they will receive a very different message about HIV/AIDS. They will learn that only deviant groups of women such as prostitutes or drug addicts are at risk. 'Normal' women who lead virtuous monogamous lives are so unlikely to 'catch' AIDS as to be for all practical purposes risk free – unless they happen to be African. One of the key themes of this chapter will be that there is growing evidence to suggest that the politically correct health promotion lobby's line on HIV/AIDS is potentially as misleading, if far less racist, sexist and homophobic, as the 'them and us' approach to AIDS adopted by certain media pundits.

In this chapter we will first explore scientific 'knowledge' about AIDS and reveal major uncertainties and controversies within the scientific community over the cause and likely cause of the heterosexual AIDS epidemic. We will then critically evaluate health promotion campaigns on HIV/AIDS aimed at women in general before focusing on two groups of women who have received special attention from the AIDS industry: prostitutes and pregnant women. The chapter will conclude with an analysis of women and HIV/AIDS which will highlight the structural factors including poverty and male power which both expose certain groups of women to a high risk of dying of AIDS and inhibit these women's abilities to adopt a behavioural strategy which might significantly reduce that risk.

Scientific "knowledge" of women, HIV and AIDS

According to a number of publications on women and AIDS, experts now know enough about the transmission of HIV and the progression from being HIV positive to having full blown AIDS to predict that millions of women worldwide are already doomed to die of AIDS. For example Fleur Sack MD in *Romance to Die For* tells her American women readers

> If you don't think AIDS is a crisis, consider the Harvard numbers. By 2000 as many as 110 million people in the world will be infected with the HIV virus. More than 40% or about 44 million of them are likely to be women.
>
> (Sack 1992: 5)

Diane Richardson's figures in *Women and the AIDS Crisis* (1987) are a little less overwhelming. She claims

> It is evidence from Central Africa ... that most seriously challenges the idea that AIDS is something women (and heterosexuals) rarely get. Studies carried out in the tropical African zone have shown that apart from infection with HIV being extremely widespread (estimates suggest that between 5 and 10 million Africans may be carrying the virus) AIDS occurs about equally in women and men ... Over the next few years thousands of African women will die from it.
>
> (Richardson 1987: 11)

Such figures about the global spread of AIDS tend to be used in the health promotion literature as a counterweight to the figures on women's deaths from AIDS in Britain and the United States. The problem with these figures from the AIDS prevention lobby's perspective is that they are rather too low to be effectively frightening. For example by the end of 1991 only 5 per cent of adults who had developed AIDS in the UK were women and only 292 total cases of AIDS had been confirmed amongst women in the UK. However Judy Bury, who presented these figures in *Working with Women and AIDS*, preceded them with the much more frightening 'fact' that according to the World Health Organization (WHO) 'Three million women are currently HIV infected and are expected to die by the year 2000' (Bury 1992: 9). Already we can see that the 'facts and figures' on AIDS are often widely varying predictions rather than hard fact. Once we begin to explore how such widely variant predictions have been calculated we soon discover a world of great uncertainty and extreme controversy. We find one set of AIDS experts convinced that current reporting of HIV and AIDS worldwide grossly underestimates the global spread of the disease, whilst another group of experts, with far less establishment clout, vehemently argue that the AIDS establishment is grossly overestimating the worldwide threat of AIDS. This controversy is only just beginning to surface in the public domain and is certainly not given any space in the AIDS prevention literature currently written for women in the UK. In order to understand this controversy we first need to look briefly at the link between HIV and AIDS.

The dominant scientific explanation of AIDS is that it is directly caused by a virus known as HIV which attacks the body's immune system. Some researchers therefore call AIDS 'HIV disease'. This simple explanation of AIDS is the model put forward by virtually all health education literature. For example, according to *HIV and AIDS: What All Women Need to Know*, produced by the North West Regional Health Authority, 'AIDS is a collection of certain symptoms and illnesses which can occur when the body's natural defences have been damaged by a virus called HIV' (Rakusen 1990: 1). This dominant view of AIDS as purely a viral disease is not however accepted by all medical experts working in the AIDS field. Originally AIDS in gay men was thought to be caused by an immunological breakdown brought on by lifestyle factors such as extensive illicit drug use and promiscuous homosexual behaviour. As Cindy Patton has recounted, however, in *Inventing AIDS* (1990) once the human immunodeficiency virus was publicly discovered in 1984 immunologists and immunological explanations of AIDS lost out to the virologists and the virus hypothesis. From then on biomedical research on AIDS was almost wholly concentrated on seeking a 'magic bullet' solution to HIV disease. The emphasis was firmly placed on developing an anti-viral vaccine – despite the enormous practical difficulties involved – and on developing and testing profitable anti-viral forms of treatment such as the drug known as AZT or Retrovir.

Despite very strong pressures from the AIDS establishment not to break rank, a significant group of dissenters within the scientific community does now exist and is beginning to make some small headway in bringing alternative scientific models of AIDS into the public domain. For example, in the USA well over 100 scientists and others have formed a 'Group for the

Scientific Reappraisal of the HIV/AIDS Hypothesis'. This group has produced a journal, *Rethinking AIDS*, in order to disseminate heretical knowledge and ideas about the cause and treatment of AIDS. Probably the most well known of these dissenting scientists is Peter Duesberg, a distinguished molecular biologist based at Harvard. Duesberg claims that 'HIV is not sufficient for AIDS' and that 'it may not even be necessary for AIDS'. He argues that the correlation between antibody to HIV and AIDS does not prove causation. Duesberg proposes that 'AIDS is not a contagious syndrome caused by one conventional virus or microbe', rather it is a new combination of conventional pathogens including viral or microbial infections and chronic drug use and malnutrition (Duesberg 1989: 755). Duesberg claims that the main reasons why AIDS has occurred in western developing countries are an increase in homosexual activity and illegal drug use in western countries since the 1960s. In Britain this view of AIDS has been publicized by Dr Gordon Stewart, Professor Emeritus of Public Health at Glasgow University who claims

> The truth is that AIDS itself is not a simple infectious disease but a complex mixture of which the HIV virus is one part. Many people believe that the cause of AIDS is solely HIV. But it is not. One of the causes of AIDS is HIV. But the onset of AIDS is hugely encouraged by high risk behaviour – by which I mean promiscuous homosexual behaviour or aberrant sex or drug taking – among people with HIV.
>
> (Stewart 1992)

Unfortunately Dr Stewart's conclusion that 'those who die of AIDS . . . facilitate their own deaths', and his implication that therefore society should not be particularly concerned or compassionate about those deaths, is likely to lead to a vehement rejection of his ideas by the health promotion establishment whose views are dominated by the admirable insistence that no one, and in particular no one group, should be in any way blamed or stigmatized as guilty AIDS carriers or sufferers.

One of the major problems with the AIDS debate to date is that the issue of the scientific cause of AIDS appears to be inextricably linked to the issue of whether or not individuals who develop AIDS are innocent victims or blameworthy degenerates. Thus gay men have understandably tended to support the view that AIDS is simply caused by a virus rather than by anything different about the sexual behaviour of gay men. Interestingly the one book focusing on women and AIDS which I have found that emphasizes the contested status of HIV as the direct cause of AIDS was published by the English Collective of Prostitutes who naturally wish to counteract the view that HIV positive prostitutes are a major cause of the spread of AIDS into the heterosexual population.

Whilst dire predictions of a massive heterosexual epidemic of AIDS in developed countries have so far been proved to be very wide of the mark, the

AIDS establishment still claims that worldwide heterosexually transmitted HIV and AIDS is out of control. According to the Panos Institute's *Triple Jeopardy: Women and AIDS* for example, HIV infection in women is set to become 'one of the major challenges to public health, health care and social support systems worldwide' (Panos Institute 1990: 11). On the grounds of such pessimistic predictions billions of dollars worldwide are being poured into research on HIV/AIDS in developing countries and into health education programmes and health promotion campaigns based primarily on the goal of promoting 'safer sex' amongst heterosexuals in developing countries. Just as the view of AIDS in the West as simply HIV disease is being increasingly challenged, however, so too some medical experts in developing countries have begun to challenge western researchers' insistence that heterosexually transmitted AIDS is devastating their populations and their economies.

The critics of the AIDS establishment view claim that HIV/AIDS is now being overdiagnosed in developing countries in several key ways. First, HIV testing may well produce a very high rate of false positives in countries where malaria is prevalent since 'people living in such regions tend to develop high concentrations of malaria antibodies in their blood which may be cross-reacting with the AIDS test, thus giving erroneous results' (Misser cited by Chirimuuta and Chirimuuta 1987). Second, routine testing for HIV is often not available in developing countries so doctors have been advised by WHO that AIDS can be diagnosed without an HIV test. The key symptoms which WHO list as symptoms of AIDS include weight loss of 10 per cent or more, chronic diarrhoea lasting longer than one month and prolonged fever lasting longer than one month. But according to the AIDS sceptics these symptoms are also key signs of chronic malnutrition and certain tropical diseases (Chirimuuta and Chirimuuta 1987). Thus more and more African women who are actually suffering from malnutrition or malaria or TB may be diagnosed as AIDS sufferers and told that they are terminally ill. According to John Rappoport in *AIDS Incorporated: Scandal of the Century*, the AIDS industry is keen to promote AIDS as a pandemic in developing countries as 'a way of substituting harmful medical drugs for what is needed: food' (Rappoport 1988). Other critics have claimed that whilst western aid agencies are prepared to spend vast sums of money re-educating 'promiscuous' Africans they are not prepared to provide basic medical care for those suffering from diseases such as malaria and TB. According to Chirimuuta and Chirimuuta (1987) the whole emphasis on Africa as a major source of the AIDS epidemic is shot through with racist assumptions about Africans, so that scientists who were quick to assume that Africans were far more promiscuous than other races never seriously investigated the possibility that AIDS was imported into Africa by white people.

A very clear example of sexism combined with racism is given by Patton (1990) who cites the abstract of a research study carried out on Nairobi prostitutes. Ninety-eight prostitutes were enrolled to assess the efficacy of the spermicide Nonoxynol-9 in preventing HIV transmission. The researchers gave half the women 'placebo vaginal suppositories' which gave them absolutely no protection against HIV. In the event more of the prostitutes using N-9 contraceptive sponges became HIV positive during the course of the research. As Patton points out it would be difficult to imagine a more unethical, anti-woman and especially anti-prostitute research protocol.

Whatever the motives of those who now claim that AIDS is running out of control in developing countries, what is all too clear is that if even a proportion of those women and children who are now being so readily diagnosed as suffering from AIDS are actually dying from other older diseases, not only may they themselves be denied cost-effective treatment, but the argument that worldwide AIDS is primarily a disease caused by unsafe heterosexual practices is significantly weakened.

The scientific debate over the exact cause of AIDS looks unlikely to be conclusively settled in the near future. Whilst the dominant view remains that AIDS is directly caused by HIV, the multifactorial model of AIDS refuses to go away. That it has completely failed seriously to challenge the HIV equals AIDS approach may well have at least something to do with the fact that the international pharmaceutical giants and all major research institutions have pinned their colours firmly to the HIV equals AIDS mast. The fact that £700 million were wiped off Wellcome's stock market value when investors responded to the results of a four year trial which found that AZT did not after all delay the onset of AIDS clearly illustrates the high financial stakes invested in the viral approach to AIDS. According to the English Collective of Prostitutes (ECP), one of the key factors behind the promotion of the view that everyone, including all sexually active women, are now at risk from AIDS is the financial gains to be made from convincing the general public that AIDS is the greatest public health threat of our time. According to the ECP

> billions of dollars in royalties made by testing people for HIV worldwide, marketing the AIDS drug AZT and researching on HIV vaccine are inhibiting those scientists, doctors and AIDS organisations who are sceptical of the HIV = AIDS theory ... Everyone faces the same choice: endorse the official version that HIV is spreading out of control and that most people who get it will eventually die of AIDS, and the money will flow – not to people with AIDS, but certainly to careers in the scientific, medical and service industry for research in HIV drugs and vaccines, and projects giving out free condoms and needles, counselling, directories, workshops etc. Question AIDS policies and their implications for health and civil rights and you won't get a penny.
>
> (Lopez-Jones 1992: 13)

In *AIDS: The HIV Myth* Jad Adams (1989) similarly emphasized the links between the emphasis on HIV as the sole cause of AIDS and profit making. He cited a 1986 investment trends analysis which estimated that the worldwide market for products to prevent, test for and treat AIDS would be worth more than three billion dollars by 1996. Adams noted that after one new drug had been tested on just 10 patients its company's shares shot up in value (Adams 1989: 203). Not only would very large sums of research money be wasted if AIDS eventually proved to be not what it now seems but many top scientists would lose their reputations. This is not to suggest that HIV has no place in the search for a full understanding of AIDS nor that the AIDS establishment is solely motivated by ulterior concerns. Nevertheless the very existence of debate and controversy over AIDS within the scientific community suggests that women should be wary of any AIDS literature which loudly proclaims to tell 'the truth' about HIV/AIDS but which actually conveys a simplistic and overconfident message that scientists now know all they need to know about the cause of AIDS and how it is transmitted.

Women, health promotion and HIV/AIDS

According to Laurence Badgley there are only approximately 200 scientists worldwide who fully understand the 'inner circle language and symbols of esoteric virology' from whence comes our understanding of HIV/AIDS. Badgley suggests that these 'priests of virology' have handed down their own interpretations of the 'higher knowledge' of nature. These few priests have informed the millions of doctors of the world as to 'how things are' with this disease called AIDS (Badgley cited by Rappoport 1988). Badgley might well have included in this equation the thousands of health promotion workers who are currently beavering away world wide to persuade heterosexuals to alter their sexual behaviour in order to prevent any further widescale spread of HIV/AIDS. In Britain both national and local campaigns against heterosexual AIDS have been aimed primarily at women. According to Tamsin Wilton (1992) there are now 'piles and piles' of safe sex literature, yet in all her years of working in the field she has only come across one leaflet aimed specifically at heterosexual men. The main emphasis within AIDS campaigns aimed at the general heterosexual population has been on encouraging women to persuade their male partners to practise safer sex by using condoms. In 1988/89 for example the Health Education Authority ran a national campaign in the mass media featuring a white youngish heterosexual couple making love (tastefully) with the heading 'AND SHE'S TOO EMBARRASSED TO ASK HIM TO USE A CONDOM'. The text underneath their heading read

> If you choose to have sex (and remember it is your choice) make sure he uses a condom. Talk to him about it today. And never feel embarrassed. Because if asking him proves awkward not asking him could prove a lot worse.

Underneath that text was the message of the whole campaign – 'AIDS: YOU'RE AS SAFE AS YOU WANT TO BE' – a message which fits totally into an individualistic model of health behaviour and links neatly with consumer choice messages in relation to health care in more general terms. Whilst at least recognizing that women may be embarrassed when asking men to use condoms, the Health Education Authority apparently assumed that women are free to exercise choice over whether or not to engage in unsafe heterosexual activities. Such an assumption completely ignores all that we know about the imbalance of power within most heterosexual relationships. As Janet Holland *et al.* have pointed out, the idea that women can freely choose to persuade men to use condoms 'ignores the nature of systematic inequalities in the social relationships between women and men' (Holland *et al.* 1990a: 4). Furthermore,

> There is a contradiction . . . between the expectations placed on women – they are assumed to be the moral regulators of sexual activity and responsible for contraception – and the imbalance in the relative power of men and women to negotiate what happens in sexual encounters.
>
> (Holland *et al.* 1990b: 1)

Holland *et al.* have also pointed out the many ways in which men use various forms of pressure including sometimes direct violence to 'persuade' women to have penetrative sex with them (Holland *et al.* 1992). Such research strongly suggests that simply teaching young women that condom use can prevent the spread of AIDS is highly unlikely to lead to a major change in women's actual behaviour. One of the advertisements in the HEA's 1988 AIDS campaign carried the headline 'I didn't want to carry condoms because I'd look easy' and then continued 'That's her excuse – what would be yours?' thus trivializing the penalties women labelled as 'easy' or 'promiscuous' can incur within a patriarchal society. Such penalties can even include being arrested for prostitution on the strength of carrying condoms. If just carrying condoms may be taken to imply a lack of sexual innocence which in turn may be seen as 'unfeminine', how much more problematic is it likely to be for a woman, particularly a younger more sexually inexperienced woman, to insist that her male partner actually uses a condom? Women are all too aware that 'men don't like using condoms' and that men assume that their sexual pleasure will be diminished through condom use. Whilst the Women, Risk and AIDS Project found that some young women were able to refuse or resist 'unsafe' sex, other young women, or the same young women on other occasions, had not felt able to insist on condom use. For example one young woman when asked 'What about using a condom?' replied 'No, he wouldn't' and added, 'No, a lot of guys don't really like them'. Holland *et al.* concluded from their research on young women, AIDS and sexual behaviour that

> it is not merely a question of informing young women about the need for safer sex and the mechanisms of condom use, they must be empowered to express their own sexual desires and to have these met in safety.
>
> (Holland *et al.* 1990b: 23)

Whilst heterosexual sexual behaviour and activity is defined primarily if not exclusively in terms of men's sexual pleasure, penetrative sex and male orgasms and while many women still reluctantly 'go all the way' because that is what their male partners want, women are hardly 'empowered' even if they manage to insist on condom use or a delay in sexual activity. Whilst the goal of non-penetrative sex being much more widely accepted as real sex is probably quite unrealistic in the foreseeable future, the goal of at least beginning to redefine male sexuality and male sexual attitudes and behaviour is not so unrealistic – but it is simply not being seriously attempted by the health education industry. For example, the North West Regional Health Authority has produced a booklet on avoiding HIV and AIDS in the 1990s which is specifically written for heterosexual men, as well as producing a sister booklet aimed at women. Unfortunately the differences between these two booklets suggest that stereotypes of male and female behaviour are simply being perpetuated rather than challenged by health education materials. For example, the book written for women has a Mills and Boon type cover featuring a fully clothed dreamy looking woman clutching a rose whereas the men's booklet has a drawing of a nude couple making love on its cover. Inside we find that a key aim of the women's booklet is 'to look at what we [i.e. women] can do to protect ourselves, our partners and our children' (Rakusen 1990) and each subsequent page is headed 'How can we protect ourselves and others?' The booklet as a whole has virtually nothing to say about sex as a pleasurable activity.

The men's booklet on the other hand makes no mention at all of men protecting anyone except themselves. Its key aim is to show the male reader 'how to enjoy the thrill of sex throughout your life without letting it be the way you become infected with HIV and without letting fear spoil your pleasure' (Roland 1990: 7). A subsequent page is entitled, 'A bit more sex, a bit less fucking'. This booklet does at least suggest to its male readers that men can gain sexual satisfaction from rubbing a woman's clitoris and making her 'groan and shudder with pleasure' but this is hardly the same as suggesting that men might begin to take more responsibility for their female partners' health and safety.

If women in Britain are finding it extremely difficult to put their increased knowledge of safer sex into practice, due at least in part to a major imbalance of power between men and women in sexual relationships, women in developing countries are often even less free to 'choose' safer sex. First, condoms may not be readily available or affordable in many developing countries. Second, many women in developing countries are both economically and culturally less equal with men than middle-class career women in the West. According to one delegate at the 1990 SWAA (Society for Women and AIDS in Africa) Conference, for example,

> Empowerment cannot happen out of nothing. In our society most women
> are illiterate which makes spreading information about AIDS very much

more difficult ... The African woman is held back by economic dependence and significant socio-cultural burdens: religious, cultural and ethnic taboos which make discussion of some issues out of the question.
(Panos Institute 1990: 32)

Women who are economically dependent on their male partners in any culture are unlikely to risk putting themselves and their children at risk of penury by demanding that their partners practice safe sex and risking that partner's anger or even desertion. One Zimbabwean woman, for example, who knew that her husband 'met with' girlfriends at beer halls and hotels and also knew that her husband might be infected with HIV and pass the virus on to her had never mentioned either the 'girlfriends' or condom use to him because she knew that either subject would 'make him very angry'. She was a well educated woman but 'as the balance of power in her marriage' lay 'with her husband she was prevented from even attempting to protect herself from HIV infection' (Panos Institute 1990: 23). Yet despite worldwide knowledge of women's inability to enforce safer sex on their dominant male partners, health educationists throughout the world continue to place their faith in educating women about safer sex, and 'empowering' them, through educational materials, to demand safer sex from their male partners.

Prostitutes and HIV/AIDS

If health educationists throughout the world have assumed that women should take primary responsibility for preventing the heterosexual spread of AIDS, one group of women in particular, prostitutes, has been accused of actually causing AIDS to spread into the heterosexual population in the first place. For example in their particularly alarmist and misleading book *Crisis: Heterosexual Behaviour in the Age of AIDS*, Masters and Johnson claim

Since prostitutes have frequent sexual contact with numerous partners, and since many prostitutes do not insist that their customers use condoms it is not hard to see how a relatively small number of AIDS infected prostitutes could infect large numbers of men. These men, not realising that they were infected could then transmit the AIDS virus to other female sex partners.

(1988: 4)

In the light of this unsubstantiated claim Masters and Johnson go on to advocate that since prostitution can no longer be regarded as a 'victimless crime' the government should crack down on prostitution, and institute a programme of mandatory HIV testing for all prostitutes. Just as some western AIDS 'experts' have blamed prostitutes for spreading AIDS amongst heterosexuals in developed countries, AIDS experts have also focused on prostitutes in developing countries as a major source of the AIDS pandemic. According to

Diane Richardson, once western researchers recognized that AIDS was not exclusively a 'gay disease' they looked for a new scapegoat: 'Women prostitutes apparently fitted the bill nicely. This has been especially true in Africa where prostitutes have been blamed for the rapid spread of infection in a number of Central African countries' (1987: 37).

Research into HIV infection amongst prostitutes has become a worldwide growth industry in its own right. Since the mid-1980s there has been a dramatic increase in sex work research and large sums of money have been spent not only in testing prostitutes for HIV antibodies but also in monitoring their behaviour and in particular their condom use. The number of research studies now being published on sex workers suggests that not only is this a lucrative field for academic researchers but that it is also an exciting and 'sexy' topic for workers whose day-to-day lives are led in rather dull ivory towers. Many of these research studies have found surprisingly low levels of HIV infection amongst prostitutes. For example, a research project designed to estimate the number of HIV positive women working as prostitutes on the streets of Glasgow found that in 1991 only 2.5 per cent tested positive. The researchers concluded

> The low prevalence of HIV infection among female street-walking prostitutes identified in this study should serve as a strong counterweight to characterisation of female prostitutes as a major reservoir of HIV infection.
>
> (McKeganey *et al.* 1992: 803)

The researchers also noted that although it was difficult to collect reliable information on condom use it was their impression that 'during most commercial sex in Glasgow a condom is used' (McKeganey *et al.* 1992: 803). Previous research studies in Europe, one in Copenhagen and one in Nuremberg had found not a single HIV positive prostitute (*The Independent*, 10 January 1987).

The AIDS establishment has assumed that sex in exchange for money is inherently unsafe sex. Just as in the nineteenth century prostitutes were seen as a major source of venereal disease so today they are accused of being a lethal source of AIDS. Prostitutes themselves however have argued persuasively that they are far less likely to indulge in unsafe sexual practices than their amateur counterparts. They have also highlighted the illogicality of assuming that HIV is more likely to be transmitted simply because sex is exchanged for money. According to the English Collective of Prostitutes, prostitute women have traditionally insisted on clients wearing condoms and are now insisting on condom use even more strongly (Lopez-Jones 1992). Their claim is borne out by researchers who have found that since the AIDS scare prostitutes in general have a very strong commitment to safer sex: 'Generally speaking clients, managers and even many governments lack the same commitment that we have seen among sex industry workers that we have worked with' (Darrow cited by Thomas 1992: 79). If any group is recklessly practising unsafe sex it is surely those male clients who offer prostitutes more money for penetrative sex without a condom. In two studies, one in Birmingham and one in Edinburgh, researchers found that approximately one-third of male clients actively sought unprotected penetration (Thomas 1992).

Whilst very little concern has been shown for prostitutes themselves who clearly risk being infected by irresponsible male clients, some researchers have concluded that prostitutes could be taught to act as health educators in relation to HIV/AIDS. For example in Australia a group of inner city prostitutes were encouraged 'to educate men about safer sex practices' (Padian 1988). In Amsterdam a prostitutes' rights group conducted a humorous campaign for prostitutes and clients with stickers saying 'Ik doe het met' – I do it with [a condom] (Panos Institute 1990). These positive approaches to prostitutes and HIV/AIDS however find little support from the right-wing press and repressive legislators who have sought – in many countries around the world – to impose new repressive laws in relation to prostitution. For example, in 1988 Newark City Council, New Jersey voted to require that all convicted prostitutes be tested for HIV but the proposal was rejected by the mayor on grounds of expense (*Washington Post*, 1 July 1988). In Madras 23 prostitutes were detained for an indefinite period after serving their detention sentence simply for having tested HIV positive (Panos Institute 1990). In Britain some police forces have displayed 'mug shots' of 'infected' prostitutes inside police stations (Lopez-Jones 1992). All such measures are highly unlikely to prevent the spread of HIV/AIDS but are highly likely to increase the public's perception of prostitutes as dangerous and diseased and to increase the risk of violent attacks on prostitutes. One English prostitute for example claims that the AIDS scare 'has lent legitimacy and credibility to anyone who wants to do violence against prostitutes ... This anti-prostitute and anti-gay epidemic has been equally dangerous to our health as AIDS itself' (Lopez-Jones 1992: 62).

Pregnant women and HIV testing

Whilst AIDS was seen to be exclusively a gay plague, gay men and AIDS activists managed to prevent policies of widespread mandatory HIV testing. They argued that testing would not actually prevent the spread of AIDS but in any case there was little public concern about AIDS when it was seen to threaten only gay men. Once it became clear however that AIDS was occurring amongst heterosexuals demands for testing programmes increased significantly and along with prostitutes, pregnant women were soon singled out for HIV testing. By 1987 mandatory or aggressive 'volunteer' testing of pregnant women had been established in a number of American states. In Britain both central government and the medical profession have resisted all calls for the mandatory testing of 'high risk' groups. In 1991 however the British Medical

Association recommended that all pregnant women should be routinely offered screening for HIV, thus demonstrating, once again, the medical profession's primary interest in women as mothers. Whilst the British government has been keen to disassociate itself from the view that HIV testing can play an important role in preventing the spread of HIV it did agree to an anonymized survey of HIV status in order to gather reliable data about the spread of the HIV virus in Britain. The two groups singled out to take part in this survey run by the Medical Research Council were patients attending genito-urinary (or STD) clinics and women attending antenatal clinics. The results of this study were published in 1991. They showed that in most of Britain only one pregnant woman in 16,000 tested HIV positive. However in inner London the figures ranged from 1 in 200 to 1 in 1,000 and in outer London and the south east the range was about 1 in 300 to 1 in 2,500. Figures from two inner London hospitals were widely cited in the press with comments such as 'a baby born to an infected mother every three weeks' and 'a ninefold HIV rise in mothers to be'. Typically figures which showed 1 in 100 heterosexual men to be HIV positive in inner London received far less press attention (Doyle 1991). Following the publication of these results the Department of Health finally announced that as soon as possible HIV screening would be offered routinely to all pregnant women in areas with high levels of HIV infection.

In 1991 an article in *The Lancet* strongly argued that counselling and testing for HIV infection should be offered routinely to all pregnant women. The author gave a number of justifications for this demand. First, 'HIV seropositive women may elect to terminate their pregnancy and contraception or sterilis-ation can be offered'. Second, 'medical care for HIV infection can be offered to seropositive women'. Third, 'pre-test and post-test counselling may educate pregnant women about methods to prevent infection with and transmission of HIV'. Fourth, 'babies born to seropositive mothers can be treated appropriately and followed for signs of development of HIV associated disease' (Barbacci et al. 1991: 710).

Let us examine each of these apparent advantages of routine HIV testing in turn. First, HIV positive women do not necessarily want an abortion and many would certainly not want sterilization. Very early studies of the risk of HIV positive mothers transmitting the virus to their unborn child suggested that approximately 50 per cent of their babies would remain infected and therefore eventually develop AIDS and die. More recent research studies, however, have produced much more encouraging results. A European collaborative study, for example, found an overall vertical transition rate in children born at least 18 months previously of only 12.9 per cent (Bury 1992: 46). When doctors assumed a 50 per cent risk of vertical transmission a number of HIV positive pregnant women were strongly pressurized to opt for an abortion. According to Sheila Henderson (1992) HIV positive women in Britain frequently report being put under pressure from health professionals to terminate pregnancy. One woman commented

I had a termination about a year ago and I was getting pressure from doctors, health advisers, all the right people giving me the wrong sort of pressure I didn't need ... I was getting a lot of pressure because I was an ex-user and I was postive. They told me I would have a child that was positive and I would go on to get AIDS.

(Henderson, 1992: 12)

Despite such pressures a significant proportion of women insisted on continuing with their pregnancy – much to the annoyance of some members of the medical profession. One HIV positive woman in the US who was admonished by her doctor for being irresponsible in becoming pregnant told him that a 50 per cent risk was the best odds she had heard since she tested HIV positive (Panos Institute 1990: 47). The option of an abortion and/or sterilisation may seem logical to doctors who have always tended to put the health and well-being of unborn babies before the well-being of pregnant women but for many HIV positive women having a child is still a life-enhancing option. According to one female obstetrician in the US the medical profession's surprise at HIV positive women choosing to have children stems from doctors' inability to see the situation from the woman's perspective: 'For many women childbearing is seen as life-affirming in the face of poverty, drug use, racism and perhaps the loss of other children to foster care or AIDS' (Mitchell cited in Panos Institute 1990: 47).

Sensitive counselling designed to help an individual woman decide whether or not she could cope with the knowledge that her child might develop AIDS might be of great help to HIV positive pregnant women. However, given the track record of antenatal clinics in relation to treating each pregnant woman as an intelligent individual who is quite capable of making up her own mind about her medical care during pregnancy and childbirth, it seems perfectly reasonable to express concern about the quality of counselling of pregnant women who test HIV positive after a 'routine' blood test.

In 1992 a commentary in the *British Journal of Obstetrics and Gynaecology* which strongly supported routine HIV testing in areas such as inner London, claimed that 'counselling is not a new or difficult skill for midwives and doctors responsible for the care of pregnant women' (McCarthy *et al.* 1992). It suggested that pre-HIV test counselling 'should be brief' and 'given by a midwife who had undergone training' (McCarthy *et al.* 1992: 868). It did not specify how comprehensive or detailed such training should be.

It is important to note the impact of undergoing a 'routine' HIV test on pregnant women who eventually test HIV negative; simply being offered a test for a disease universally regarded as fatal will inevitably cause stress and anxiety in most pregnant women. Moreover, given women's own accounts of how difficult they have found it to resist other 'optional' tests during pregnancy, we must at least speculate that women who refuse the test may well be labelled as 'irresponsible' by antenatal staff.

The claim that once doctors know a pregnant woman is seropositive they can offer her 'appropriate' medical care looks rather thin once we accept that modern medicine has yet to find any effective form of treatment for asymptomatic HIV positive patients. Now that a large long term clinical trial of AZT has demonstrated its ineffectiveness in delaying the onset of AIDS in HIV subjects (Concorde Coordinating Committee 1994), all that doctors can offer is lifestyle counselling. Whilst good counselling can clearly help an HIV positive woman come to terms with her extremely difficult position, it is at least arguable that her own health and well-being would have been far higher if she had remained ignorant of her HIV status, since there is clearly a high psychological price to be paid for being given what amounts to a death sentence.

Clearly the main motive behind calls for increased HIV testing of pregnant women is to reduce the spread of the infection to both male partners and crucially 'innocent' unborn children. Critics of HIV testing policies have repeatedly pointed out, however, that they are a very poor method of preventing spread of the virus and that in particular a negative test result is likely to encourage 'unsafe' sexual activities when the key aim of health prevention programmes should be to encourage everyone, regardless of their current HIV status, to practice 'safer' sex (see Hepburn 1992). Moreover routine voluntary HIV testing amongst pregnant women will do virtually nothing to prevent vertical transmission unless those women who test positive are pressurized or even forced to terminate their pregnancies, a policy which seems increasingly unjustifiable given the relatively low risks of vertical transmission in Europe. In 1994 it was claimed that the results of an unpublished study suggested that zidovudine (AZT) given to HIV positive mothers during pregnancy reduced the transmission of HIV to the fetus (Lipsky 1994). If this result is confirmed it could well lead to increased pressure on pregnant women to accept HIV testing and to then take AZT for the sake of their unborn child if they proved HIV positive and did not wish to have an abortion. The key problem with this prospect is that AZT is known to produce such bad side effects that it seriously reduces the quality of life of those taking it (Lipsky 1994). Once again, therefore, pregnant women may be pressurized to put their own well-being aside for the sake of the fetus.

The final claim, that knowing the HIV status of the mother will improve the medical care given to HIV positive babies again does not stand up in the light of the lack of any effective treatment for asymptomatic HIV positive babies. Once such babies develop AIDS symptoms they can presumably receive appropriate treatment regardless of whether they were previously known to be HIV positive.

Overall therefore the case for offering routine HIV testing to pregnant women would appear to be thin whilst the dangers inherent in such a programme are all too clear. Not only have a number of HIV positive pregnant women already experienced very strong pressure to accept an abortion but a woman's HIV status may well play an even greater role in determining her reproductive rights in the future. As more and more women are pulled into 'artificial' reproduction programmes such as IVF and GIFT they will also be pulled into 'routine' HIV testing and those who test positive will find it extremely difficult to gain treatment. One infertility specialist has already publicly stated that it would be unethical for him to treat an HIV positive infertile couple. How big a leap would it be from this position to a demand that all HIV positive women should be sterilized to protect the health of future generations? Fortunately many British doctors, who are now treating HIV positive women with great sensitivity, would strongly resist such a demand but the whole history of women's constant fight to defend and extend their reproductive rights strongly suggests that women should not complacently accept routine HIV testing of pregnant women as a wholly benign form of screening.

Women, poverty and HIV/AIDS

Whilst most health promotion workers have adopted a model of HIV/AIDS which assumes that there are no high or low risk groups but only high risk and low risk behaviours, a growing number of AIDS experts are beginning to acknowledge that heterosexual AIDS is primarily a disease of poverty. Whilst the health promotion industry continues to pour resources into an individualistic behaviour modification approach to the prevention of HIV/AIDS, it is becoming increasingly clear that women's greatest risk of AIDS lies not in their own ignorance or wilful disregard of their own health, but in their economic disadvantage and relative poverty. In the United States in the 1980s AIDS was a disease which affected white middle-class men. By the 1990s AIDS was killing primarily poor black and Latino women and men (Panos Institute 1990).

In the UK the majority of women who have so far been found to be HIV positive are injecting drug users or partners of injecting drug users (Bury 1992). These drug users live predominantly in deprived inner city areas. It is not the illegal drugs themselves which infect women but the sharing of contaminated equipment and/or unprotected sex with HIV positive drug users. In New York a crack epidemic in the poorest neighbourhoods has led to an epidemic of sexually transmitted diseases including AIDS among women who sell their bodies in order to raise money to buy crack. Non-drug users may wish to argue that women who use illegal drugs are responsible for their own high risk of HIV infection. However this common view of women drug users as an undeserving group ignores the strong links between illegal drug use and poverty. As Don Edwards has pointed out, illegal drug use worldwide is at least in part a reflection of 'frustration and anger of marginalised and impoverished populations seeking escape through mood-altering drugs' (Edwards cited by Panos Institute 1990: 7).

Not only do the conditions of poverty create an environment in which unsafe individual behaviour is more likely to occur, they also make it far more difficult for conventional health promotion programmes to succeed. According to Edith Springer, if the majority of women who are most vulnerable to HIV infection are struggling daily to meet their own survival needs and those of their children,

> trying to get them to focus on health promotion and AIDS prevention is a difficult task. It is a great fear of theirs, yet they feel helpless to do anything about it. In order to do real AIDS prevention work we have to first meet these women's survival needs.
>
> (Springer 1992: 40)

If this argument holds true for women living in the US – one of the most affluent countries in the world – how much more true will it be for poor women living in developing countries?

Not only do women living in poverty face a far higher risk of HIV infection and AIDS than affluent women, they are also likely to receive very limited medical and social care if they do develop AIDS. In 1989 the United States spent an estimated five billion dollars on AZT therapy, mainly for those with good health insurance, whilst black women living in inner city ghettoes who developed AIDS tended to receive very inadequate and fragmented treatment, care and support (Panos Institute 1990). In Britain the existence of the NHS provides, in theory at least, a much more egalitarian health care system, but HIV positive women have nevertheless experienced hostility and discrimination from some health and welfare professionals and a lack of interest in their health care needs from the medical research establishment. One British HIV positive woman has expressed her anger at the way she and other HIV positive women have been treated: 'anger at the lack of appropriate or accessible services, anger at needs not being recognised or met' (Thomson 1992: 137). She has also expressed her anger at 'the thousands and thousands of pounds' spent on

> dodgy research and flying people halfway around the world club class to present the results of their work. They should instead be spending research money on looking into the important issues that we still know so little about – like how the virus affects women's bodies for instance.
>
> (Thomson, 1992: 137)

Women affected by HIV/AIDS have called for far more research into HIV/AIDS to include women subjects as well as men (e.g. Thomson 1992). Unfortunately the history of AZT and indeed the history of so many 'magic bullet' solutions to modern diseases strongly suggests that the real long term solution to AIDS is unlikely to lie with the pharmaceutical companies and the medical research which they fund and support. Whilst both governments and the drugs industry continue to pour resources into finding a magic vaccine which will prevent HIV infection and/or a magic pill which will prevent HIV turning into full blown AIDS, relative poverty and deprivation are increasing in Britain and so too are all the economic and social conditions which leave certain women so vulnerable to the risk of AIDS. Yet which Health Minister or health education spokesperson would publicly announce that Child Benefit and Income Support were being significantly increased as an anti-AIDS initiative? It is far more politically expedient for governments to focus on individualistic health education campaigns against AIDS which cost relatively little and convey the message that everyone must look after their own health in this as in all other areas. It is far more capitalism-compatible to allow pharmaceutical companies to offer extremely expensive forms of anti-AIDS therapy to terminally ill patients rather than to create good employment prospects and healthy exciting environments for young people living in deprived inner cities where the heterosexual AIDS risk is greatest.

Discussion

There is no doubt that an increasing number of women in Britain are becoming HIV positive and that a growing, but still very small, number of women are personally affected by AIDS. Whilst not wishing to put any woman's life at risk by underestimating the threat of AIDS it is essential to put this risk into perspective. The health promotion/AIDS industry insists that the currently low female death rate from AIDS is misleading since what really counts is the number of women infected with HIV. As we have seen, however, measuring the extent of the AIDS risk by using HIV statistics is controversial. A growing number of AIDS experts are beginning to publicize their argument that being HIV positive is not invariably a death sentence. Some experts now claim that if HIV positive individuals do not engage in any immunosuppressant activities such as using recreational drugs and if they do everything possible to strengthen their immune systems they may well live long and healthy lives (Gavzer 1990). Because this alternative view is sometimes expressed by those who wish to blame certain groups in society for 'indulging' in 'dangerous' behaviour such as 'promiscuous' sexual activity, many AIDS workers tend to dismiss this view out of hand. Yet if we logically distinguish the hypothesis that there may be co-factors, such as drug taking, which increase the risk of HIV converting to full blown AIDS from any moralistic or punitive attitudes towards drug users or gay men, we may discover new, more optimistic approaches towards those who are already HIV positive. We accept that smoking causes lung cancer but surely we do not therefore argue that all smokers deserve to die from lung cancer? Yet when HIV/AIDS is debated far too many experts on both sides of the political divide fail to distinguish between possible causes of a medical syndrome and the quite separate issues of blame and stigmatization of AIDS sufferers. Taking seriously the view that the link between HIV and AIDS may be less clear cut and simple than the now dominant model of AIDS does not in any way imply a 'them and us' punitive response to AIDS sufferers. Nor does it imply that women who are not 'promiscuous' or injecting drug users can happily ignore all messages about safe sex. HIV is certainly not the only major health risk to women which is sexually transmitted. Long before the AIDS panic women have suffered the penalties of 'unsafe' sex including infertility, cervical cancer and unwanted pregnancies. Condoms and other barrier methods of contraception have many advantages for all sexually active women if only they had the power to persuade their male partners to accept them. Any attempts to empower young women to carry and use condoms are certainly to be welcomed however limited their effects. This does not mean however that young women should be frightened into suppressing their own sexual desires by alarming and potentially highly misleading information about the rapid global spread of HIV and AIDS amongst women. Many AIDS workers are no doubt disseminating alarming predictions of an AIDS epidemic amongst women with the best possible intentions, but it is at least worth wondering whether the AIDS establishment and the pharmaceutical companies in particular may be exaggerating HIV/AIDS figures in order to create an ever-growing global market for their anti-AIDS products including health education, condoms and anti-AIDS drugs.

The evidence to date suggests that despite the massive efforts of the health promotion/AIDS industry sexually active British women have not whole-heartedly adopted safer sex practices (Wilson 1992). Mass education campaigns can effectively increase knowledge about a particular form of risky behaviour, but they have proved far less effective in actually changing that behaviour. Early campaigns against AIDS launched by national governments tended to fall into the same old trap. The British government's 'tombstones and icebergs' AIDS campaign was almost universally regarded as both alarming and ineffective. In Australia the government launched the 'grim reaper' campaign which portrayed AIDS as a scythe carrying skeleton in medieval garb who indiscriminately bowled over human skittles – men, women and children – in an underworld bowling alley. An evaluation of that campaign found that it dramatically increased public awareness of AIDS but that it also spread fear and panic amongst those who in reality were extremely unlikely to be HIV positive. Moreover after the TV campaign discrimination against HIV positive people increased but the fear which had been spread about AIDS did not prompt 'appropriate changes in behaviour' (Winn 1991).

Since these early national campaigns much more sensitive and well-thought out local initiatives have been developed to promote behavioural change in relation to HIV risk. In Britain local 'outreach' programmes have been devised to protect particular groups of women such as sex workers and intravenous drugs users (Wilson 1992; MacIver 1992). Such initiatives have had some limited successes, particularly where AIDS workers have fully involved the women themselves in the setting up and running of the projects. AIDS workers themselves however are all too aware that they are usually working in an extremely hostile environment. One safer sex counsellor who has worked with illicit drug using women has commented

> the work of HIV prevention is a far more challenging task than we initially imagined ... most of the women with whom I have worked have internalised their powerlessness which often leaves them with feelings of despair, defeatism and fatalism ... In this context the modification of sexual behaviour to reduce the risk of HIV infection is a formidable undertaking.
>
> (Wilson 1992: 115)

Providing illegal drug users with clean equipment as well as counselling and advice is a step towards protecting them from the risk of HIV/AIDS. Similarly, ensuring that sex workers have an adequate supply of condoms is useful. By themselves however even these practical prevention measures are highly unlikely to counteract the effects of socioeconomic deprivation. Just as many single mothers living in poverty continue to smoke despite knowing all too well the health risks involved, so too will sex workers who are desperate for money occasionally put themselves at risk of HIV infection, as will poor drug addicts who are desperate for their next fix. Poverty and extreme relative deprivation do not, of course, totally remove a woman's ability to choose a healthy lifestyle but they certainly make such a choice very difficult. This already widely accepted view applies just as much to HIV/AIDS as to other late twentieth-century diseases, despite the initial view of AIDS as a new and unique form of illness. It therefore no longer makes sense to attempt to combat HIV/AIDS as though it were either a totally indiscriminate disease or a punishment for wickedness. Heterosexual AIDS is primarily a disease of poverty and deprivation. Until that causal link is publicly accepted and tackled poor women will increasingly be at risk from dying of AIDS regardless of how many resources are thrown into AIDS prevention programmes and the search for a 'cure' for AIDS.

If it is now essential to make overt links between poverty and women's risk from AIDS it is also crucial to explore the relationship between HIV/AIDS, the AIDS establishment and the increasing scrutiny and control being exercised over women's sexuality. Traditionally women's sexuality has been closely and often violently controlled by their male partners. Women's sexuality has also been subjected to patriarchal control by a male dominated medical profession. During the 1970s and 1980s some feminists began tentatively to explore and debate the meaning of sexual autonomy and desire for women. Liberal feminists discussed the myth of the vaginal orgasm whilst radical feminists totally rejected all forms of heterosexuality in favour of political and personal lesbianism (see, for example, Leeds Revolutionary Feminist Group, 1982). Even women who had absolutely nothing to do with the feminist movement began to demand, from the late 1960s onwards, greater sexual freedom and greater sexual satisfaction. Women as a group thus began very slowly and painfully to challenge and even reject a centuries old patriarchal ideology of women as sexually passive and sexually prone. Then in the mid-1980s the AIDS panic began. Very quickly the fragile notion that women could engage in sexual activity primarily for their own guilt free pleasure was dealt a double blow. On the one hand right-wing moralists warned women that only the virtuously monogamous would be saved from the cesspit of AIDS. On the other hand 'right on' AIDS workers, including some feminists, warned all sexually active women that unless they covered virtually every orifice with latex or cling film they would be guilty of taking a totally irresponsible risk with their long term health and life. The drive towards 'safer sex' now seems more or less universal and unstoppable. Even lesbians, who are widely acknowledged to have an absolutely negligible risk of contracting HIV from their sexual practices, have been advised to use dental dams to prevent any transmission of body fluids during sexual activity (Richardson 1989). By 1990 there had been only two cases reported worldwide of women becoming infected with HIV through sex with another woman (in both cases the sexual activities involved included the exchange of blood). Yet one writer in *Spare Rib* condemned as 'criminal' the fact that dental dams, unlike condoms, are not freely available in public places such as pubs and clubs. She also found the absence of specific information for lesbians on the risk of HIV/AIDS an indictment on every HIV and AIDS agency (Montsho 1991). Lesbians who are intravenous drug users may be at risk from AIDS and certainly need to know how to protect themselves and their partners. Lesbians who wish to get pregnant using artificial insemination also need information on the risk of contracting HIV through this means. Nevertheless it does seem sad that women whose sexual practices are clearly very 'low risk' are still being urged by some AIDS experts to consider 'rubber dams' and other safety paraphernalia which clearly problematize sex and create certain barriers to intimacy.

Not only has the fear of AIDS created a demand for no-risk sex regardless of either the financial or personal price to be paid, it has also created a whole new band of pseudo-medical experts who now police women's sexual activities. Many AIDS workers who are appalled by right-wing moralists' demands that women should return to being virtuous and monogamous happily instruct women with long and technical lists of the dos and don'ts of new safer sex practices (see Richardson 1989). These instructions will inevitably create a whole new range of female anxieties and inhibitions in relation to sex.

According to the German feminist Sabine Marx (1990), the messages about safe sex now being pumped out by the AIDS establishment and even by some feminist AIDS experts serve to strip sexuality of all feelings. She claims that much of the safer sex literature portrays women as 'in essence nothing but orifices' in a rather similar way to pornography. She asks women whether they want their bodies to be seen as 'the new risks' and whether they want further state control over their 'bodily orifices', whether they want all their sexual activities categorized by self-appointed experts into dangerous and non-dangerous categories? Perhaps women just have to accept that sex is – as it always has been – a risky, even potentially dangerous, activity for them. It may not be possible for women to be sexually active and remain 100 per cent safe from HIV/AIDS. This does not mean that women should act recklessly but they may need to challenge at least some of the frightening messages which now descend upon them from a potentially oppressive AIDS establishment. Women who wish to avoid ever-increasing official controls over their most intimate lives may have to create a woman-centred anti-AIDS movement based not on fear and spurious expertise/authority but on women's own needs and desires. Yet this crucial enterprise is unlikely to even get off the ground if we continue to allow the so-called fight against AIDS to be dominated worldwide by an AIDS establishment which claims to be the fount of all knowledge on HIV/AIDS but which promotes safer sex from within an almost exclusively patriarchal and profit/career oriented paradigm.

9

CONCLUSION

A recently graduated student of mine, with whom I was discussing the writing of this book informed me that many students read only the conclusion to a book on the grounds that it will usually contain a summary of all the author's key points. For the benefit of any such readers, as well as for all those who have actually read the preceding chapters but would still like to know what overall conclusions the author draws from them, this conclusion will present the book's five key themes. They are: first, that modern medicine is less beneficial to their health than most women assume; second, that medical interventions frequently impose both physical and psychological harm on individual women as well as inflicting social harm on women as a group; third, that women health care consumers lack the information they require to make wise choices about their treatment; fourth, that very strong vested interests play a crucial role in determining the health care system's priorities and overall direction; fifth, that women's health could best be improved by spending less on modern medicine and more on other areas of social policy.

The benefits of modern medicine

The evidence presented in this book has demonstrated over and over again that modern medicine is far less beneficial to women's overall health and well-being than most people assume. This conclusion does not just apply to so-called curative or 'high tech' health care such as the treatment of breast cancer, it applies equally to medical screening and to many health promotion activities.

Undoubtedly, some medical interventions do provide effective answers to women's health problems. Some types of treatment appear to be effective nearly all of the time, whilst others appear to work at least some of the time. It is therefore virtually impossible to give categorical answers to individual women wondering whether or not to accept a particular type of treatment. For example, whilst the critics have made a very good case for the view that breast and cervical cancer screening programmes save far fewer women's lives than their most ardent supporters would have women believe, the critics have not proved, and in most cases do not even try to prove, that such programmes save no women's lives at all (Chapter 6). Similarly, whilst critics of psychotropic drugs have presented a very convincing case that they are overprescribed to women and are often ineffective, some women suffering from severe anxiey or depression have testified that these drugs were of great benefit to them, at least in the short term (Chapter 5). Large numbers of menopausal women have also loudly sung the praises of HRT even if it has never been scientifically proven to be be an anti-ageing device (Chapter 4). Finally, whilst some health education messages aimed at women appear to be based on very flimsy scientific or epidemiological evidence, others are at least giving women accurate information even if other factors prevent women from responding to it (Chapter 7). Whether or not women living in poverty 'choose' to smoke, there is little argument about the dangers such smoking poses to their health and longevity. The significant conclusion in relation to the effectiveness of vast amounts of health care currently consumed by women is not therefore that it is all useless but that its benefits tend to be greatly oversold by many of those involved in providing it.

Health care providers have been slow to admit that particular health care products or interventions have been proven to be ineffective. The British medical profession is known for its less interventionist approach than, for example, the American medical profession. Doctors in Britain are also known for maintaining a healthy scepticism in relation to new 'wonder drugs' and 'breakthrough' surgical techniques. For example, in the 1950s British doctors were much less enthusiastic than American doctors about the effectiveness of the hormonal treatment of Diethylstilboestrol (DES) for threatened miscarriages. Twenty years later young women in Britain were far less at risk of developing vaginal cancer as a consequence of their mothers taking DES during pregnancy than their American counterparts (Taylor 1979). In the 1990s British doctors appear similarly cautious about prescribing the new wonder drug Prozac which is being taken by millions of Americans as a mood elevator. Moreover, in recent years doctors working within the NHS have begun to adopt new systems of medical audit which promise to ensure, on paper at least, that ineffective forms of treatment and unacceptable individual practice will be more quickly detected and deleted. Yet despite British doctors' relative scepticism and increased policing of their own practices, ineffective medical practices continue to flourish. In recent years we have witnessed an unfortunate tendency for one type of ineffective medical treatment to be gradually phased out only to be replaced by a new intervention which spreads almost like wildfire before strong doubts about its effectiveness grow. For example, radical mastectomies are finally being phased out as a treatment for early breast cancer as more and more surgeons begin to accept the evidence – which has existed for decades – that they do not save or even prolong women's lives (see Jennett 1986). Rather than simply do less in response to breast cancer however, the medical profession is constantly experimenting with new cocktails of treatment, for example trying out new types of chemotherapy in combination with surgery and sometimes radio-therapy. Some of these experimental forms of treatment may prove to be more effective than mastectomies in prolonging the lives of breast cancer patients. Far too often however, experimental forms of breast cancer treat-ment have been hailed as a 'breakthrough' long before clinical trials have been completed or thoroughly evaluated. Having failed to treat successfully existing breast cancers, the medical profession is now moving towards treating women even before they exhibit very early signs of the disease. Enthusiasts for the drug Tamoxifen for example, are strongly advocating its use as a preventative form of medicine in young women with very high genetic risk of breast cancer, despite concerns about the drug's long term safety. Some doctors are even offering double mastectomies to young women who appear to have a particularly high risk of developing breast cancer. Given the failure of mastectomies to cure existing breast cancer this new form of preventative medicine could be seen as medical imperialism at its most rampant (see Chapter 6).

The drive to intervene even after medical intervention has been shown to be relatively ineffective can also clearly be seen within modern obstetrical practice. Fetal monitoring, for example, is now used routinely in virtually all obstetric units despite relatively strong evidence of its almost complete ineffectiveness (Chapter 2).

'High tech' curative health care appears to have taken on such a strong momentum that evidence of its ineffectiveness merely leads to a change of technique rather than a move back to less interventionist forms of care. Even very low tech forms of health care provision are not immune to the trend of ever-expanding in the face of evidence that their previous activities failed to achieve their goals. For example, when scientific research began to suggest that simply avoiding saturated fats would not save people's lives, health promotion workers, instead of giving up their emphasis on the need for everyone to adopt a healthy low fat diet, simply modified their precise advice a little and, without pausing for breath, continued to lecture women about their unhealthy dietary habits. The key reasons for this drive towards ever increasing health care activity will be explored later, the main conclusion to be reached at this stage is simply that much of the 'curative' treatment, diagnostic screening and health promotion advice consumed by women in the late twentieth century is far less effective in terms of improving their health than virtually all of those providing it lead women to believe.

The harmful effects of modern medicine

Very few women are killed by medical treatment. Nevertheless many routine forms of medical intervention do carry very small short term and long term risks of mortality. For example, it has been estimated that the risk of dying from taking the contraceptive pill a for non-smoker under the age of 35 is 1.3 per 100,000 (Guillebaud and Law 1987). One woman in Britain has now died as a direct result of undergoing IVF treatment although again statistically this risk is extremely small. This death hit the headlines but the far greater number of women who die each year from taking an overdose of prescribed drugs, particularly anti-depressants, is not newsworthy. Such deaths are immediate and relatively easy to quantify but women taking long term medical treatment also face less immediate risks of increased mortality. For example, there is now a quite well established link between long term use of HRT and an increased risk of endometrial and breast cancer (Chapter 4). As far as hormonal forms of contraception are concerned, medical experts still cannot decide conclusively whether they do increase women's overall risks of breast or cervical cancer, but some research evidence has certainly been less than reassuring (Chapter 1).

Whilst the risk of death associated with most modern medical interventions is undoubtedly extremely small and in many cases not conclusively proven, the risks of unpleasant or uncomfortable physical side effects from a whole range of medical interventions are both widespread and clearly documented. Many women taking prescribed hormonal preparations of various types have reported significant physical side effects including headaches, vaginal irritation and heavy or irregular bleeding (to name but a few) (see Chapter 1). Women undergoing routine obstetrical interventions such as inductions or artificial rupturing of membranes have reported experiencing pain over and above that experienced naturally in childbirth. Some women who have been screened for cervical or breast cancer have been shocked to discover that a test promoted as painless can actually be experienced as very painful by a minority of patients. Women vary in their response to a whole range of medical interventions. Some women will experience pain or discomfort whilst other women experience no physical side effects or pain whatsoever. Moreover some women may believe that the benefits to them of a particular form of treatment or diagnostic technique outweigh the physical costs. Most women do not appreciate however, being told by their doctor that the strong pain they experience during a particular medical procedure is either 'minor discomfort' or even 'imaginary'. Nor do they always agree with the medical profession's definition of a 'minor' side effect. Irregular or heavy bleeding may seem relatively trivial to a male doctor prescribing Depo Provera, but it is not always experienced as such by a woman who has not been adequately warned that such side effects are relatively common.

If the physical side effects of medical interventions are difficult to measure objectively, the negative psychological effects of medical diagnoses and treatments may be even less amenable to objective scientific measurement. Moreover it is particularly difficult to prove that a depressed mood, for example, is directly related to a particular drug or treatment rather than the illness being treated or indeed to a woman's life in general. Nevertheless, meticulous research by social scientists has produced strong evidence of women's negative emotional responses to a whole range of routine medical interventions. Even some proponents of cancer screening programmes now accept the strong body of evidence documenting the serious psychological distress which a preliminary positive test result imposes on women.

Whilst anxiety may be a natural response to any type of screening for cancer, other forms of psychological distress may be induced by a range of drugs which doctors commonly prescribe to women. Despite an initially sceptical response many doctors now accept that some women feel depressed as a direct result of taking an hormonal contraceptive. Similarly, the medical profession now recognizes that women who have taken tranquillizers for any length of time may experience acute psychological distress if they attempt to stop taking these drugs too abruptly. Finally we should emphasize that even good medical advice may produce an adverse psychological reaction in some women. For example, a pregnant women who smokes may experience increased stress during pregnancy if faced with a barrage of medical advice on the dangers her smoking poses to her unborn child. Ironically this stress may actually contribute to an increase in her tobacco consumption. Women are experts at feeling guilty. If they do manage to control any guilt over their own 'unhealthy' habits they will almost certainly suffer guilt if they cannot afford to provide their families with the healthy lifestyle now advocated by their medical advisers.

According to Illich, modern medicine is not simply physically and psychologically disabling on an individual level, it also creates 'social iatrogenesis'. Illich claims that social iatrogenesis occurs when 'suffering, mourning and healing outside the patient role are labelled as a form of deviance' and 'the malignant spread of medicine ... turns mutual care and self medication into misdemeanours or felonies'. Illich also argues that

> iatrogenic medicine reinforces a morbid society in which social control of the population by the medical system turns into a principal economic activity. It serves to legitimize social arrangements into which many people do not fit ... People who are angered, sickened and impaired by their industrial labour and leisure can escape only into a life under medical supervision and are thereby seduced or disqualified from political struggle for a healthier world.
>
> (1977: 51)

I have cited Illich at some length because so much of his argument relates directly and distinctly to women as health care consumers. Illich's critique can be applied to women in three distinct ways. First, feminists who have suggested that women should 'suffer' or 'mourn' at various times in their lives without turning to modern medicine for a 'cure' or a 'crutch' have been derided as extremist or even 'dotty' by the popular media. When Germaine Greer (1992) argued, for example, that menopausal women should give up attempting to look attractive for men and go through a period of mourning for their lost youth before emerging into a sexless serene old age she was generally regarded as eccentric. Second, feminists who have attempted to create a demedicalized women's health movement based on self-help have faced strong opposition from the medical profession or certain leading sections of it. Carol Downer, an American feminist who helped to set up self-help clinics for women in California, was actually arrested in 1972. Her crime was that she had inserted yoghurt into a woman's vagina without a medical licence, a crime of which she was eventually found not guilty (Dreifus 1978). Third, as well as exercising monopolitic power over the provision of health care, the medical profession plays a major role in giving advice to women about how to live their lives. To feminists much of this advice is a form of patriarchal control over women as a group. This patriarchal control has been exercised by male doctors for well over one hundred years.

From the late nineteenth century to the mid-twentieth century women have been treated with surgery for deviating from their alloted female roles. As late as the 1970s, for example, some psychiatric textbooks were recommending lobotomies to enable women to cope with their marriages (Showalter 1987). By the 1990s psychosurgery was far less commonly perfomed on women but it was still advocated by some psychiatrists as a treatment of last resort. Much more ubiquitous in the late twentieth century is the use of psychotropic drugs to dampen down women's distress and an endless stream of medical advice to women on how to be good wives and mothers. Pregnant women in particular have been singled out for particularly vehement medical advice designed to curb if not eliminate all their 'dangerous' habits. Ironically women who cannot get pregnant naturally have also been subjected to intrusive medical advice. Some women, for example, have been told by their GPs that they cannot be selected for scarce infertility treatment unless and until they improve their drinking, eating and smoking habits.

Young unattached women do not necessarily escape lectures from their doctors. Young women who have been unfortunate enough to catch a sexually transmitted disease from a male partner have reported being given a moral lecture from their doctor about their sexual behaviour (see Furedi, 1994). Older women suffering from stress and exhaustion whilst attempting to combine a full time job with the traditional caring role have been advised by doctors to give up or cut down paid work rather than let down their husbands and children by neglecting their housewife role (Roberts 1985).

Overall evidence presented in this book has clearly suggested that modern medicine tends to medicalize a range of problems which women face primarily because of their unequal position in society. Some doctors even appear to blame women themselves for health problems which are caused primarily by poverty, male domination or racial discrimination. A classic example of this is those doctors who talk about the irresponsibility of poor young women who 'who get themselves pregnant' as though neither young men, nor the education system, nor a society which fails to offer these women interesting and viable alternatives to motherhood had any influence on teenage pregnancy rates. Whilst women's problems are thus individualized and medicalized, the medical profession and the health care industry more generally can be regarded as playing at least some part, if not a major role, in disabling women as a group and distracting them from the fight for political, social and economic solutions to their collective problems.

Lack of accurate information

Women today have access to far more information about medical matters than at any other time in history. Medical experts of all kinds write accessible articles in women's magazines and in newspapers. Official health organizations such as the Health Education Authority produce leaflets and booklets on a whole range of women's health issues and doctors in general are more informative and open than they used to be. If a woman fails to get all the information she wants from an official source she can buy a book on women's health or on a particular woman's health problem from any major bookshop. She can even choose to consult books on health and health care written from an explicitly feminist perspective. Yet despite this apparent wealth of information on health matters, evidence presented in this book has strongly indicated that unless women read a range of learned medical journals for themselves they will be unlikely to receive a wholly accurate picture of the effectiveness and side effects of any particular type of medical intervention or treatment.

There are at least three reasons why women still fail to receive a full and accurate account of the costs as well as the benefits of modern medicine. First, doctors themselves may not be fully aware of the risks attached to certain medical treatment. Many initial clinical trials of drugs have excluded women as research subjects, sometimes for no apparent reason (Horton 1994). Some pharmaceutical companies have claimed that women are excluded from many drugs trials because of the particular risks to women who might become pregnant whilst testing a new drug. Whatever the main reason for their exclusion, the consequence is that the information needed to evaluate the safety of a new drug specifically in relation to women frequently does not exist. However, even if information is available not all GPs will be fully cognizant with it themselves, particularly as most GPs receive more information about new drugs from drugs companies than from official sources (Audit Commission 1994). Information from drug representatives will inevitably stress a drug's efficacy and safety rather than stressing its potential risks. GPs may not therefore be in the best position to give their patients full information about the potentially negative or even dangerous side effects of a particular drug even if they believed that patients should receive such information. In some cases doctors may even be convinced of the efficacy of a particular type of treatment despite strong research evidence of its ineffectiveness. Supporters of ECT appear to fall into this category (see Chapter 5).

Second, some doctors still appear to believe that their female patients could not cope with too much information about a particular type of treatment, for example, breast cancer patients rarely seem to be given totally accurate information about all the treatment options available to them. Some cancer specialists have argued for example, that it would be unfair and unkind to expect a woman with breast cancer to cope with complicated and often depressing information about the efficacy of different types of treatment. Third, the media tends to disseminate a remarkably positive view of the efficacy of modern medicine. Miraculous medical breakthroughs which will positively transform the lives of women are routinely headline news in the popular press. The contraceptive pill, HRT, Tamoxifen, cervical screening and IVF are just a few of the modern medical discoveries hailed as of great benefit to women by a somewhat naive media. In recent years the British media have been extremely critical of the resourcing and management of the NHS. Riddles such as 'How many NHS employees does it take to change a lightbulb?' are commonplace. Meanwhile a minority of journalists have sometimes questioned doctors' attitudes towards women and have even queried the benefits of certain medical treatments such as tranquillizers and HRT. Nevertheless the main criticism of Britain's health care system by the mainstream media has focused on women's lack of access to the best and most expensive medical care available rather than on the issue of whether even the best and most expensive medical care lives up to its promises. A good example of this trend was a *Panorama* programme on breast cancer treatment broadcast in March 1994. The programme exposed the lottery of care and treatment faced by women with breast cancer in Britain. It implied that women could be dying unnecessarily because of lack of breast cancer specialists. Too many surgeons, the programme claimed, were dabbling in breast cancer treatment and failing to offer their patients the best mix of diagnosis and up-to-date effective treatment. What this programme did not do was to challenge the assumption made by both patients and breast cancer specialists that the best treatment on offer is a very effective treatment for this disease.

Women who ask their own doctors lots of questions about their health care, women who read widely about health issues in the popular press and women who seek out official health promotion literature may all assume that they are relatively well-informed health care consumers. Evidence presented in this book, however, suggests that much of the information women health care consumers receive is strongly biased towards an overly optimistic view of the efficacy and safety of modern medicine. Without a major shift in this information imbalance, the government's current emphasis on consumerism within the health care system will only serve to reinforce an already distorted demand for a medicalized solution to every health problem women experience. A very few privileged women may gain access to less biased health care information but even they are unlikely to have either the time or the inclination to undertake their own academic research into the hidden world of medical doubt, uncertainty and disagreement about the costs and benefits of modern medical interventions.

Vested interests in health care

Perhaps the most fundamental theme to emerge from the preceding chapters is that women's health care, even within the NHS, is primarily determined by the interests of the providers of health care rather than the needs of women themselves. This bias occurs in at least three key ways. First, most health care providers are primarily concerned to defend and improve their own employment prospects including their working conditions. Second, many medical specialists and researchers seek professional recognition, status and prestige. Third, pharmaceutical and medical equipment companies are very closely entwined with all modern health care systems and are driven primarily by the goal of large profits rather than the ethic of service to the patient. Let us examine each of these three factors in more detail.

The NHS is one of the biggest employers in the world. It provides direct and indirect employment for over a million people. Its labour force is divided into a very large group of low paid workers and a relatively small group of highly paid professional workers. The majority of low paid, low status workers in the health care industry are women. They have virtually no control over their area of work and cannot exert any influence over the type of health care provided, apart perhaps from partly determining the quality of some of its basic day-to-day services such as cleaning and catering. At the top of the NHS hierarchy are the managers and health professionals who are predominantly male. (In 1991 only 15.5 per cent of NHS consultants and 18 per cent of NHS general managers were female; Department of Health 1994). These top employees play a key role in determining the nature of hospital and community based health care services. If they are deemed successful in their jobs they can earn very high salaries and enjoy a wide range of occupational perks. Top acute specialists are no longer the only health care providers to enjoy high incomes within the NHS. Since 1990 the number of very highly paid managers within the NHS has soared. Some community-based health care workers also enjoy high salaries. In February 1994 the popular press reported the scandal of a senior health official who had resigned as Chief Executive of Health Promotion Wales (a government funded quango) after admitting an affair with a colleague during official trips abroad. The scandal apparently was the possibility that he had fiddled his expenses. No one seemed to think that his annual salary of £80,000 plus endless trips to foreign conferences might be scandalous in itself. Although most of those employed in the ever-growing health promotion industry earn far less than £80,000 per annum, basic health promotion officers can now earn up to £25,000 per annum. Given such salaries one would hardly expect many health promotion officers to argue publicly that much health education may cause more harm than good. Similarly, one would not expect many consultant obstetricians to publicize the view that much modern obstetrics may be both ineffective and harmful. The hidden agenda of maintaining employment for health care providers has also been noted by Vernon Coleman in relation to the breast cancer screening programme. He noted that at the time the government launched a breast cancer screening programme which would need the services of many radiologists to read the mammograms, it just so happened that, for several years, Britain had been training 32 radiologists more than it needed each year. Coleman commented, 'The new breast screening programme will help to mop up the glut of potentially unemployed radiologists' (1988: 174). In fact medical screening programmes do not just provide work for all those involved in administering, carrying out and checking the screening tests. They also create extra work for the acute health care sector by creating many more 'patients' in need of 'curative' treatment.

It would be quite untrue to suggest that doctors, or indeed radiologists, played a key role in developing mass screening programmes primarily in order to improve their own employment prospects. Most GPs, for example, have increased their cervical screening activity only as a response to financial incentives laid down by the Department of Health. Nevertheless individual GPs can now increase their own, or at least their practice's, income by increasing certain types of health care activity. For example GPs can earn extra income by providing contraceptive services for their female patients. With the recent creation of fundholding general practices and trust hospitals, direct links between health care activity and income have been greatly increased within the NHS, moving it slightly closer to the fee-for-service health care systems which have an in-built bias towards overtreating patients. Senior managers in the newly created trust hospitals, including acute specialists, appear to have gained particular freedom to improve their own working conditions. According to Bartlett and Le Grand's analysis of trust hospitals it is crucial to understand the paradox that although trusts are non-profit making organizations, 'their principal objective is profit-maximisation' (1994: 69). Bartlett and Le Grand explain this apparent paradox by pointing out that those at the top of trust hospitals will personally benefit from generating large surpluses either by directly increasing their incomes or by improving the quality of their working conditions (Bartlett and Le Grand 1994). They speculate that trust hospitals may well grow in a fashion which will increase the incomes and working conditions of the decision-making group as much as possible. Such growth would probably be capital intensive rather than an increase in staff in order to restrict 'the number of workers among whom any perks or residual income may be divided'. Trusts might thus develop 'as providers of specialised high quality services using predominantly capital-intensive technologies'. According to Bartlett and Le Grand, 'this would still be medicine primarily in the interests of the doctor rather than medicine in the interests of the patient' (Bartlett and Le Grand 1994: 70). It would certainly be the type of high technology medicine which this book has suggested frequently imposes least benefit and most harm on women and their health.

Whilst some trust managers may be primarily interested in maximizing their own incomes, the medical profession as a whole is clearly not solely, or even primarily, interested in personal monetary gain. Many doctors may be more interested in their public status than their private income. According to Bryan Jennett

> For many doctors conspicuous private consumption (e.g. a Rolls Royce) has been replaced as a status symbol by conspicuous public consumption. To be seen to be developing and expanding new technological procedures signals success.
>
> (Jennett 1986)

In 1976 an article in the *New England Journal of Medicine* identified a new disease, 'CAT fever'. The article claimed, tongue in cheek, that

> The predominant symptom appears as a feverish impulse to own, operate, exploit or write about what has been known as computerized axial tomography (CAT). CAT fever has reached epidemic proportions and continues to spread among physicians.
>
> (cited by Taylor 1979)

In the 1980s a very similar article could have been written about ultrasound fever or electronic fetal monitoring fever. Both these 'high tech' machines have undoubtedly contributed to the job satisfaction and status of obstetricians but whether they have contributed anything positive to the health and well-being of pregnant women and their babies remains far from clear.

Whilst practising doctors within the acute health care sector appear to seek job satisfaction by using the latest medical technology, medical researchers seek to be at the cutting edge of medical innovation and discovery. They too often appear to seek not so much high private incomes as well resourced public research laboratories. They also seek the public status and prestige to be gained from being the first to make some kind of medical breakthrough. The very public row between French and American research scientists over the discovery of the 'AIDS virus' illustrated the importance that researchers attach to being publicly recognized as 'coming first'. Medical research does not just take place in laboratories. At some point patients must be involved in testing a new drug or surgical technique. At this point the interests of patient and researcher may well conflict. We noted in Chapter 3, for example, how women suffering from infertility were originally used as research guinea pigs in experimental infertility treatment programmes which had yet to produce a single live healthy baby. Yet many of these women appeared not to have been fully informed of the experimental nature of their treatment.

Whilst medical specialists and researchers may well include treating patients effectively as one of the key measures of their job satisfaction, the key goals of medical equipment manufacturers and pharmaceutical companies appear to be much further removed from the ethic of giving primacy to patients' well-being. A number of exposés of the workings of international pharmaceutical giants have clearly documented the extent to which the drive for profits tends to override all other concerns (see, for example, Melville and Johnson 1983). Whilst the general public may still wish to regard the NHS as an institution with quite different goals from those of private industry, all modern health care systems, including the NHS, are so closely entwined with the private manufacturers of medical products that it is virtually impossible to separate out the various interests involved. For example, according to the Audit Commission (1994), 'Hormone replacement therapy (HRT) is an example of a treatment which, while often beneficial, has mushroomed in cost following publicity in popular magazines'. In other words according to the Audit Commission the increased prescribing of HRT is primarily due to 'more informed patients' or increased patient demand for treatment. As we noted in Chapter 4, however, pharmaceutical companies have used women's magazines to promote HRT directly to potential patients whilst at the same time targeting GPs with both soft and hard sell promotions for HRT. Meanwhile a growing number of specialists have adopted the view that the menopause is a treatable deficiency disease, and this view is now being taught to younger GPs. We thus have a combination of factors all leading to increased prescribing of HRT in Britain. Some GPs may argue that it is women themselves who are demanding HRT. Some women may claim that HRT has been pushed on them by their doctors. Meanwhile pharmaceutical companies are strongly encouraging both doctors and patients to see HRT as the solution to all women's menopausal problems, primarily in order to boost their profits from this range of drugs.

Women in Britain may assume that doctors working within the NHS are far less likely to be completely entwined in the worst excesses of profit driven prescribing than their counterparts in fee-for-service health care systems. Doctors in the NHS do indeed prescribe far fewer drugs than most other European doctors. For example, in 1989 the average French person received 38 prescriptions compared to the British 7.6 (Audit Commission 1994: 4).

Nevertheless GPs' prescribing costs within the NHS continue to rise despite government attempts to hold them in check. In 1992–93 the total cost of GP prescribing was £3,309 million. Whilst over 40 per cent of drugs prescribed by GPs are now cheaper generic brands, new patented drugs continue to generate very large profits for their manufacturers. In the early 1990s, for example, pharmaceutical companies heavily promoted newer types of anti-depressants known as SSRIs as being safer than the older tricyclics which are now relatively cheap. These newer types of anti-depressants cost on average 10 times more for an equivalent dose, yet research evidence supporting claims that they are much safer is inconclusive (Audit Commission 1994).

The exact profits which pharmaceutical companies make from selling their wares to the NHS are a state secret. Government negotiations with these companies over the price of prescribed drugs are complicated by the state's dual role. On the one hand it aims to ensure that drugs are purchased by the NHS at a reasonable price but on the other hand it also aims to promote a strong and profitable British pharmaceutical industry. As the Audit Commission has commented, with some restraint, 'the aims of promoting a strong efficient British pharmaceutical industry and securing good value for the NHS do not always sit easily together' (Audit Commission 1994: 5). As Michael Moran has pointed out,

> Pharmaceuticals remain one of the few important industries where the United Kingdom, a manufacturing economy in decline for over a century, still retains a significant world presence. Indeed whereas most British industries have been sinking out of sight in world rankings, British pharmaceutical companies like ICI and Glaxo have moved into the top ranks in the last two decades.
>
> (Moran 1994)

A capitalist industrial state like Britain can hardly afford to undermine the profits and international status of one of its few remaining viable industries. A similar dilemma faces the government in relation to the NHS purchase of high technology medical equipment. On the one hand it may wish to curb the spread of machines such as electronic fetal monitoring machines whose efficacy has yet to be proven. On the other hand it may welcome the boost to employment such purchasing provides.

Overall, whilst the NHS does reduce the scope for exploitation of patients in a number of important ways, such as paying surgeons a salary rather than a fee for every operation they perform, it is clear from much of the evidence presented in this book that women's health care is primarily shaped by the vested interests of a whole range of health care providers. Far from being an island of disinterested public service surrounded by a sea of profit oriented private markets, the NHS is very much entwined with the private sector. The title of this book was chosen as a reminder to women health care consumers that rather than being similar to a church the NHS today more resembles a garage (Klein 1993). Women who take their car into a garage for a service or repairs are probably all too aware that the mechanics therein may exaggerate the car's problems and the extent of repairs needed in order to maximize their own income. Yet women as health consumers all too often trust health care providers to put all other interests aside apart from that of providing the best patient care. Women might question the medical advice and treatment they receive more often if they were more aware of the links between that advice and treatment and the large personal and company gains made by many of those working in, for, or alongside the NHS; gains moreover which are highly dependent on a continuing supply of female consumers of mainstream medical wares.

Improving women's health

Modern medicine undoubtedly plays a role in maintaining women in good health. Even modern medicine's most vigorous critics usually find at least a few aspects of modern medicine which they accept as effective and beneficial. Most critics of modern obstetrics, for example, accept that a Caesarean section is occasionally a life saving operation. Similarly, most critics of the rising tide of hysterectomies do not claim that these operations are always completely unnecessary. They can, for example, prevent early uterine cancer from developing into a more invasive and life-threatening form of cancer. In virtually every chapter of this book examples have been given of women who have clearly benefited from medical intervention. This book does not claim, therefore, that all modern medicine is a totally ineffective and damaging response to women's health needs and problems. It does suggest, however, that overall the benefits of modern medicine to women have been greatly oversold and that alternative, more effective responses to women's health needs have been totally overshadowed by the mainly unsubstantiated claims of high technology medicine. In this final section three alternative answers to women's health problems will be briefly outlined. They are first, a redistribution of income designed to lift significant numbers of women out of severe relative poverty; second, a major increase in the social and practical support given by the state to women in their caring roles and to women in need of long term care; third, a new emphasis by the health promotion industry on men's responsibility for the health and well-being of their female partners. All these policy options can be defined as forms of primary prevention in contrast to the activities of modern medicine which revolve around the diagnosis and treatment of existing health problems.

There is an ever-growing body of evidence linking women living in poverty to greatly increased risks of morbidity and premature mortality. For example nearly two-thirds of Britain's one million lone mothers are officially defined as living in poverty and researchers have found that lone mothers report themselves to be in poorer health more often than parents in couples and more often than lone fathers (Millar 1992). A large national survey of people's health and lifestyle carried out in the mid-1980s found that lone parenthood had an 'extremely disadvantageous effect' on women's health, especially their psychosocial health (Blaxter 1990).

Another large group of women who are very vulnerable to poverty are women over pensionable age. More than twice as many women as men live in or on the margins of poverty in old age. Amongst those over 80 the ratio is approximately 5 to 1 (Walker 1992). Women over the age of 60 tend to occupy hospital beds for longer periods than men and although they are hospitalized less frequently than elderly men, they visit their GP significantly more often than men and have particularly high rates of minor mental disorders (Kane 1991). Since most people associate old age with increased ill health such figures may be assumed to reflect natural tendencies towards health problems in later life. Given the clear links between poverty and ill health amongst young people, however, it would be logical to assume that the severe relative poverty suffered by so many elderly women has a very detrimental effect on their health and well-being.

The precise relationship between poverty and women's ill health is not easy to determine. Those on the right of the political spectrum tend to argue that many women deemed to be living in poverty choose unhealthy lifestyles and spend their incomes unwisely on unhealthy items such as junk food and cigarettes. However, a number of researchers have documented the extent to which women living in poverty, particularly women with children, cannot afford to adopt healthy lifestyles and often continue unhealthy behaviours such as smoking in response to the stresses imposed on them by their very poor circumstances (see Chapter 7). In any case the national health and lifestyle survey concluded that adopting healthy behaviours made little difference to women's health if they were living in poor environments (Blaxter 1990).

According to Quick and Wilkinson (1991) the key reason why relative poverty in Britain is linked to ill health is the impact it has on social support, social participation and self-esteem, all of which are closely related to health. Quick and Wilkinson argue that higher overall standards of living may improve the material circumstances of the poor in an absolute sense but that if the relative gap between the poor and the rest of society is not narrowed the poor will continue to suffer the health-denying effects of relative deprivation. The only way to improve the health of the nation according to Quick and Wilkinson's thesis will be to improve the relative incomes of the poorest groups in society. If we apply Quick and Wilkinson's thesis specifically to women it would mean significantly improving the relative incomes of women, in particular lone mothers, female pensioners and women who are full time 'unpaid' carers. The exact means of achieving such a redistribution need not be spelled out here but it would clearly involve higher taxes on the better off, including relatively affluent women. It could also involve reducing expenditure on relatively ineffective forms of health care such as routine antenatal visits and using the resources saved to boost the income of women living in poverty – perhaps more specifically poor pregnant women. Unfortunately any such shift in social policy would be highly unlikely to win significant public support. Even women living in poverty might oppose any reductions in health care spending since they have been taught since childhood that high technology medicine saves lives. Despite such strong beliefs empirical evidence clearly supports the view that increased financial support would improve the health and well-being of women living in very poor circumstances far more effectively and efficiently than any increased expenditure on high technology health care or even on health promotion activities.

One of the most damaging consequences to women of severe relative deprivation is the social isolation which so often accompanies it. Lone mothers living on income support and elderly women living solely on state pensions are two groups that are particularly vulnerable to minor mental disorders such as depression and anxiety. More practical support from the state might well help to relieve this very common form of health problem. For example, many lone mothers are strongly in favour of the provision of more affordable and available public child care facilities which would enable them to go out to work (Bradshaw and Millar 1991). Not only would paid work provide them with an additional income, it could also improve their self-esteem and increase their rate of social participation. Similarly, many elderly women living alone could greatly benefit from more social contact which could be provided by enhanced community care services. Yet whilst expenditure on acute health services has risen significantly in recent years, despite misleading cries of 'cuts' from prominent health care providers (see Department of Health 1994), the government has resolutely refused to fund any major increase in state nursery provision. The government has also failed to fund the expansion of community care services needed to support adequately the increasing numbers of frail elderly people living in the community. Not only do inadequate support services isolate frail elderly women living on their own, they also leave younger women carers to bear incredibly heavy loads of community care without adequate support. The frail elderly and their carers, however, do not appear to have the same political influence over resource allocation as shroud waving acute specialists who insist that patients will die if more resources are not poured into high technology medicine.

If women's health is put at risk because of their relative economic deprivation in our society and the lack of adequate state support for their caring activities, it is also endangered by their relative powerlessness in relation to men. The medical profession and politicans frequently refer to the problem of unwanted pregnancies among teenage girls as though pregnancy was a state which these girls achieve all by themselves. Similarly doctors frequently warn women that cervical cancer is linked to their promiscuous behaviour. Only very rarely are women's male partners mentioned as in any way sharing the responsibility for unwanted pregnancies or the spread of cervical cancer. The focus on persuading women to use condoms in recent health promotion campaigns simply continues this trend of holding women primarily responsible not only for their own health but for the health and well-being of their male partners and children. At its most extreme this ideology blames women for putting the health and safety of themselves and their children at risk by failing to leave violent male partners. If the medical profession and health promotion workers began to take more seriously men's responsibility for the health of the nation, they might begin to focus on how to persuade men to do far more to protect the health of their partners and children. They might, for example, launch a health education campaign designed to improve men's awareness of their role in preventing unwanted pregnancies and sexually transmitted diseases such as chlamydia (which can cause female infertility) and HIV/AIDS. They might also persuade men not to smoke whilst their partners are pregnant. However even if the health promotion industry did turn its attention to men's roles in this way, all the evidence presented in this book suggests that a major shift in men's behaviour could not be achieved using current health promotion techniques. Much wider social change will undoubtedly have to occur before men accept much greater responsibility for the health and well-being of their female partners.

The way forward

Since the mid-1970s the women's health movement in Britain and the USA has played a key role in critically evaluating modern medicine's impact on women's health and well-being and in demanding action for change. Many women health activists have devoted enormous amounts of time and energy to creating an alternative model of health care provision based on the feminist principles of egalitarian sharing of health knowledge and woman centred advice and treatment (see Foster 1989). Not only has the women's health movement provided women with an alternative model of the delivery of health care, it has also encouraged some doctors within mainstream medicine to become more open and less authoritarian within the doctor–patient relationship. Whilst any such changes may well improve women's experiences of health care it is crucial to note that improvements in the relationship between doctors and their female patients do not by themselves create a significantly more effective health care system. Women suffering from the sickening effects of economic deprivation, racial harassment or sexual violence will not be 'cured' by more sympathetic doctors nor by yet more resources being poured into medical technology. Those wishing to improve the overall health and well-being of women in our society should not be seduced by the extremely influential messages of the health care industry. The medicalization of all women's problems is disabling and disempowering. Women need to fight for change without, as well as within, the health care system, since any significant long term improvements in women's health are unlikely to occur until women get the economic and social changes needed to create a truly healthy environment within which all women can flourish.

REFERENCES

Action on Smoking and Health (ASH), Working Group on Women and Smoking (1993) *Her Share of Misfortune*. London: Action on Smoking and Health.

Adams, J. (1989) *AIDS: the HIV Myth*. London: Macmillan.

Alcohol Concern (1988) *Women and Drinking*. London: Alcohol Concern.

American Medical Association, Council on Scientific Affairs (1983) Estrogen replacement and the menopause. *Journal of the American Medical Association*, 249(3), 359–61.

American Psychiatric Association (1987) *Diagnostic and Statistical Manual of Mental Disorders (DSM III R)*, 3rd edn. Washington DC: American Psychiatric Association.

Amos, A., Jacobson, B. and White, P. (1991) Cigarette advertising and coverage of smoking and health in British women's magazines. *The Lancet*, 337, 93–96.

Anderson, P. (1991) Alcohol as a key area, in R. Smith (ed.) *Health of the Nation: the BMJ View*. London: British Medical Journal.

Armstrong, L. (1991) Surviving the incest industry. *Trouble and Strife*, 21, 29–32.

Arnold, M. (1985) Where obstetrics fail. *Midwife, Health Visitor and Community Nurse*, 21, 346–7.

Ashton, H. and Golding, J. F. (1989) Tranquillisers: Prevalence, predictors and possible consequences. Data from a large United Kingdom Survey. *British Journal of Addiction*, 84(5), 541–6.

Association for Improvements in Maternity Services (AIMS) (1991) *Supplementary Memorandum submitted by the Association for Improvements in Maternity Services in House of Commons Health Committee Second Report Vol. II Minutes of Evidence*. London: HMSO, 471–99.

Audit Commission (1994) *A Prescription for Improvement: Towards More Rational Prescribing in General Practice*. London: HMSO.

Bailar, J. (1985) When research results are in conflict. *New England Journal of Medicine*, 313(17), 1080–81.

Barbacci, M., Repke, J. T. and Chaisson, R. E. (1991) Routine prenatal screening for HIV infection. *The Lancet*, 337, 709–11.

Barnes, M. and Maple, N. (1992) *Women, Mental Health and Social Work*. Birmingham: Venture Press.

Barrett, J. F., Jarvis, G. J., MacDonald, H. N., Bucham, P. C., Tyrrell, S. N. and Lilford, R. J. (1990) Inconsistencies in clinical decisions in obstetrics, *The Lancet*, 336, 549–51.

Bartlett, W. and Le Grand, J. (1994) The performance of trusts, in R. Robinson and J. Le Grand (eds) *Evaluating the NHS Reforms*. Hermitage: Policy Journals.

Bastias, G. (1992) Contraception news: DP use in inner city areas. *Women's Health Newsletter*, 15, 12.

Bates, G. (1988) The American fertility society and industry: A vital relationship. *Fertility and Sterility*, 50(3), 398–9.

Beardow, R., Oerton, J. and Victor, C. (1989) Evaluation of the cervical cytology screening programme in an inner city health district. *British Medical Journal*, 299, 98–100.

Berer, M. (1989) Contraception, in A. Phillips and J. Rakusen (eds) *The New Our Bodies: Ourselves*. London: Penguin Books.

Bergkvist, L., Adami, H., Persson, I., Hoover, R. and Schairer, C. (1989) The risk of breast cancer after estrogen and estrogen-progestin replacement, *New England Journal of Medicine*, 321(5), 293–7.

Bewley, S. and Bewley, T. (1992) Drug dependence with oestrogen replacement theory. *The Lancet*, 339, 290–91.

Billingsley, J. (1987) Taking the toys from the boys. *AIMS*, Winter, 5.

Birtchnell, J. (1988) Depression and family relationships. *British Journal of Psychiatry*, 153, 758–69.

Blackwell, R. *et al.* (1987) Are we exploiting the infertile couple? *Fertility and Sterility*, 48(5), 735–9.

Blaxter, M. (1990) *Health and Lifestyles*. London: Tavistock/Routledge.

Bolsen, B. (1982) Question of risk still hovers over routine prenatal use of ultrasound. *Journal of the American Medical Association*, 247, 2195–7.

Bowen-Simpkins, P. (1988) Contraception by age group. *The Practitioner*, 232, 15–20.

Brackbill, Y., Rice, J. and Young, D. (1984) *Birth Trap*. St Louis: The Morby Press.

Bradshaw, J. and Millar, J. (1991) *Lone Parent Families in the UK*. Department of Social Security. Research Report No. 6. London: HMSO.

Breggin, P. (1993) *Toxic Psychiatry*. London: Fontana.

Brown, G. W. and Harris, T. O. (1978) *Social Origins of Depression: A Study of Psychiatric Disorders in Women*. London: Tavistock.

Brown, P. (1993) Breast cancer: a lethal inheritance. *New Scientist*, 18 September, 34–37.

Bruch, H. (1974) Perils of behaviour modification in treatment of anorexia nervosa. *Journal of the American Medical Association*, 230, 1419–22.

Bryan, B., Dadzie, S. and Scafe,S. (1985) *The Heart of the Race*. London: Virago.

Buchan, H., Johnstone, E., McPherson, K., Palmer, R. L., Crow, T. J. and Brandon, S. (1992) Who benefits from electroconvulsive therapy? *British Journal of Psychiatry*, 160, 355–9.

Bucher, H. and Schmidt, J. (1993) Does routine ultrasound scanning improve outcome in pregnancy? Meta-analysis of various outcome measures. *British Medical Journal*, 307, 13–17.

Bunkle, P. (1984) Calling the Shots? The international politics of Depo-Provera, in R. Arditti, R. Klein and S. Minden (eds), *Test-Tube Women*. London: Pandora Press.

Bury, J. (1987) Unwanted pregnancy and abortion, in A. McPherson (ed.) *Women's Problems in General Practice*. Oxford: Oxford University Press.

Bury, J. (1992) Women and the AIDS epidemic: some medical facts and figures, in J. Bury, V. Morrison and S. McLachlan (eds.) *Working with Women and AIDS*. London: Routledge.

Butler, E. (1984) What do we know about ultrasound? *Childbirth News*, 5(2), Spring.

Caplin, R. (1993) in Pembroke, L. R. (ed.) *Eating Distress: Perspectives from Personal Experience*. Chartridge. Chesham: Survivors Speak Out.

Carson, S. A. (1988) Sex selection: The ultimate in family planning. *Fertility and Sterility*, 50, 16–19.

Chamberlain, J., Coleman, D., Ellman, R. and Moss, S. M. (1988) First results on mortality reduction in the UK Trial of early detection of breast cancer. *The Lancet*, II, (8608), 411–16.

Chamberlain, J., Moss, S. M., Kirkpatrick, A. E., Mitchell, M. and Johns, L. (1993) National Health Service breast screening programme results for 1991–2. *British Medical Journal*, 307, 353–6.

Chapman, S. (1979) Advertising and psychotropic drugs: The place of myth in ideological reproduction. *Social Science and Medicine*, 13A, 751–64.

Charles, N. and Kerr, M. (1986) Eating properly, the family and state benefit. *Sociology*, 20(3), 412–29.

Charlton, A. (1990) Women and smoking, in N. Pfeffer and A. Quick (eds), *Promoting Women's Health*. London: King Edward's Hospital Fund for London.

Chesler, P. (1972) *Women and Madness*. New York: Avon Books.

Chilvers, C., McPherson, K., Peto, J. and Pike, M. C. (1989) Oral contraceptive use and breast cancer risk in young women. *Lancet*, 1 (8645), 973–82.

Chirimuuta, R. C. and Chirimuuta, R. J. (1987) *AIDS, Africa and Racism*. Brety: Derbyshire.

Chomet, J. and Chomet, J. (1990) Cervical screening in general practice a 'new' scenario. *British Medical Journal*, 300, 1504–6.

Cohen, G. R. and Duffy, J. C. (1992) Alcohol-drinking and mortality from diseases of circulation, in J. C. Duffy (ed.) *Alcohol and Illness: The Epidemiological View*. Edinburgh: Edinburgh University Press.

Cohen, R. (1988) *Psychiatric Consultation in Childbirth Settings*. New York: Plenum Medical.

Coleman, V. (1988) *The Health Scandal*. London: Mandarin.

Concorde Coordinating Committee (1994) Concorde: MCR/ANRS randomised double-blind controlled trial of immediate and deferred zidovudine in symptom-free HIV infection. *The Lancet*, 343, 871–881.

Consensus Development Conference (1986) Consensus development conference: treatment of primary breast cancer. *British Medical Journal*, 293, 946–7.

Conway, J. (ed.) (1988) *Prescription for Poor Health*. London: IFC, Maternity Alliance, Shalc and Shelter.

Coope, J. (1987) Menopause, in A. McPherson (ed.) *Women's Problems in General Practice*. Oxford: Oxford University Press.

Cooper, W. (1979) *No Change*. London: Arrow Books.

Cooperstock, R. and Lennard, H. (1986) Some social meanings of tranquilliser use, in J. Gabe and P. Williams, *Tranquillisers, Social, Psychological and Clinical Perspectives*. London: Tavistock.

Corea, G. (1985) The reproductive brothel, in G. Corea *et al. Man Made Women*. London: Hutchinson and Co.

Corea, G. (1988) *The Mother Machine*. London: Women's Press.

Corob, A. (1987) *Working with Depressed Women*. Aldershot: Gower Publishing.

Cox, B. D. *et al*. (1987) *The Health and Lifestyle Survey: Preliminary Report*. London: The Health Promotion Research Trust.

Crossen, R. (1953) *Diseases of Women*, 10th edn. London: Henry Kimpton.

Cunningham, M. (1992) Why midwives should scan. *Midwives Chronicle and Nursing Notes*, February, 36–7.

Curran, V. and Golombok, S. (1985) *Bottling It Up*. London: Faber and Faber.

Currie, E. (1989) *Lifelines*. London: Sidgwick and Jackson.

Daly, M. (1978) *Gyn/Ecology*. Boston, MA: Beacon Press.

Davey, B. (1988) Social side of cancer. *Marxism Today*, March, 30–3.

Day, N. (1991) Comments on abstaining for foetal health. *British Journal of Addiction*, 86(9), 1057–61.

Dean, M. (1992) Health, but not for all. *The Lancet*, 340, 166.

Department of Health (1992) *The Health of the Nation and You*. London: HMSO.

Department of Health (1994) *Departmental Report*. Cm 2512. London: HMSO.

Department of Health and Social Services (DHSS) (1986) *Breast Cancer Screening* (the Forrest Report). London: HMSO.

Dobson, J. (1992) Thirty years' hard labour. *Health Service Journal*, 12 March, 10.

Dominian, J. (1990) *Depression*. London: Fontana.

Douglas, G., Hebenton, B. and Thomas, T. (1992) The right to found a family. *New Law Journal*, 142, 6547, 488–90.

Dowie, M. and Johnston, T. (1978) A case of corporate malpractice and the Dalkon Shield, in C. Dreifus (ed.) *Seizing Our Bodies*. New York: Vintage Books.

Doyal, L. (1979) *The Political Economy of Health*. London: Pluto Press.

Doyal, L. (1987) Infertility – a life sentence? Women and the National Health Service, in M. Stanworth (ed.) *Reproductive Technologies*. Oxford: Blackwell.

Doyle, A. (1991) HIV/AIDS News. *Women's Health and Reproductive Rights Information Centre Newsletter*, 12 July, 25.

Doyle, C. (1991) The unjust cost of parenthood. *The Daily Telegraph*, 23 July.

Dreifus, C. (ed.) (1978) *Seizing Our Bodies*. New York: Vintage Books.

Duesberg, P. (1989) Human immunodeficiency virus and acquired immunodeficiency syndrome: correlation but not causation. *Proceedings of the National Academy of Sciences of the USA*, 86, 755–64.

Duffy, J. C. (1992) Alcohol consumption and liver cirrhosis, in J. C. Duffy (ed.) *Alcohol and Illness: The Epidemiological View*. Edinburgh: Edinburgh University Press.

Duffy, S. W. and Sharples, L. D. (1992) Alcohol and cancer risk, in J. C. Duffy (ed.) *Alcohol and Illness: The Epidemiological View*. Edinburgh: Edinburgh University Press.

Dunne, F. (1988) Are women more easily damaged by alcohol than men? *British Journal of Addiction*, 83(10), 1135–6.

Durward, L. (1988) *Poverty in Pregnancy*. London: Maternity Alliance.

Dyer, C. (1992) 16 year old's refusal of treatment overruled. *British Medical Journal*, 305, 76.

Edwards, R. *et al*. (1989) Letter to the editor: Benefits of in-vitro fertilisation. *The Lancet*, 11, 1328.

Ehrenreich, B. and English, D. (1979) *For Her Own Good*. London: Pluto Press.

Ethics Committee of the American Fertility Society. (1986) Ethical considerations of the new reproductive technologies. *Fertility and Sterility*, 46(3), Supplement 1.

Ettinger, B. and Grady, B. (1993) The waning effect of postmenopausal estrogen therapy on osteoporosis. *The New England Journal of Medicine*, 329 (16), 1192–3.

Ettorre, E. (1992) *Women and Substance Use*. Basingstoke: Macmillan.

Expert Maternity Group (1993) *Changing Childbirth*. London: HMSO.

Fallowfield, L. J., Hall, A., Maguire, G. P. and Baum, M. (1990) Psychological outcomes of different treatment policies in women with early breast cancer outside a clinical trial. *British Medical Journal*, 301, 575–80.

Faulder, C. (1989) *The Women's Cancer Book*. London: Virago.

Felson, D. *et al.* (1993) The effect of postmenopausal estrogen therapy on bone density in elderly women. *The New England Journal of Medicine*, 329 (16), 1141–6.

Fielding, J. (1987) Smoking and women. *The New England Journal of Medicine*, 317 (21), 1343–5.

Firth, H. V., Boyd, P. A., Chamberlain, P., Mackenzie, I. Z., Lindenbaum, R. H. and Huson, S. M. (1991) Severe limb abnormalities after chorian villus sampling at 56–66 days' gestation. *The Lancet*, 337, 762–3.

Forrest, F., Florey, C., Taylor, D., McPherson, F. and Young, J. A. (1991) Reported social alcohol consumption during pregnancy and infants' development at 18 months. *British Medical Journal*, 303, 22–6.

Foster, P. (1989) Improving the doctor/patient relationship: A feminist perspective. *Journal of Social Policy*, 18 (3), 337–61.

Francis, A. (1986) It can be done – but at what cost? *New Generation*, June, 21.

Francome, C. (1986) The fashion for Caesareans. *New Society*, 17 January, 100–1.

Francombe, C. (1989) *Changing Childbirth*. London: Maternity Alliance.

Freeman, C. P. and Kendell, R. (1986) Patients' experiences of and attitudes to electroconvulsive therapy. *Annals of the New York Academy of Sciences*, 462, 341–52.

Freeman, R. (1991) The idea of prevention: A critical review, unpublished paper presented at British Sociological Association Annual Conference, March.

Fuller, P. (1991) Race to beat cancer. *Daily Express*, 13 September, 1.

Furedi, A. (1991) Doctors and morals. *New Woman*, April, 2–16.

Gabe, J. (ed.) (1991) *Understanding Tranquilliser Use*. London: Tavistock/Routledge.

Gangar, K. and Key, E. (1991) Presentation of menopausal symptoms, *Well Woman Team*, 1(4), 8–9.

Garner, L. (1979) *The NHS: Your Money or Your Life*. Harmondsworth: Penguin.

Gavzer, B. (1990) Life after AIDS. *What the Doctors Don't Tell You*, 1 (7), 1–4.

Godlee, F. (1992) Regions coordinate family planning services. *British Medical Journal*, 304, 401.

Goldman, H. (1992) *Review of General Psychiatry*. 3rd edn. London: Prentice-Hall.

Goldman, L. and Tosteson, A. (1991) Uncertainty about postmenopausal estrogen – time for action not debate. *New England Journal of Medicine*, 325 (11), 800–2.

Graham, H. (1987) Women's smoking and family health. *Social Science and Medicine*, 25, 47–56.

Graham, H. (1993) *Hardship and Health in Women's Lives*. Hemel Hempstead: Harvester Wheatsheaf.

Greenwood, J. (1987) Depression, in A. McPherson (ed.) *Women's Problems in General Practice*. Oxford: Oxford University Press.

Greer, G. (1984) *Sex and Destiny*. London: Picador.

Greer, G. (1992) *The Change: Women Ageing and the Menopause*. London: Penguin.

Gregson, E. H. (1985) Barrier Methods, in N. Loudon (ed.) *Handbook of Family Planning*. Edinburgh: Churchill Livingstone.

Guillebaud, J. (1985) Combined oral contraceptive pills, in N. Loudon (ed.) *Handbook of Family Planning*. Edinburgh: Churchill Livingstone.

Guillebaud, J. and Law, B. (1987). Contraception, in A. McPherson (ed.) *Women's Problems in General Practice*. Oxford: Oxford University Press.

Guthrie, C. (1990) 'A long term follow-up study of patients with anorexia nervosa'. Unpublished MSc Thesis, University of Manchester.

Hadley, J. (1987) The case against Depo-Provera, in S. O'Sullivan (ed.), *Women's Health: A Spare Rib Reader*. London: Pandora.

Hale, A. S., Proctor, A. W. and Bridges, P. K. (1987) Clomipramine, Tryptophan and Lithium in combination for resistant endogenous depression: Seven case studies. *British Journal of Psychiatry*, 151, 213–7.

Haney, A. (1987) What is efficacious infertility therapy? *Fertility and Sterility*, 48 (4), 543–4.

Hayman, S. (1993) *The Family Planning Association Guide to Contraception*. London: Harper Collins.

Health Committee (1991) *Second Report on Maternity Services*. London: HMSO.

Health Education Authority (HEA) (1989) *NHS Breast Screening: The Facts*. London: HEA.

Health Education Authority (HEA) (1991) *Pregnancy Book*. London: HEA.

Helman, C. G. (1986) 'Tonic', 'Fuel' and 'Food': social and symbolic aspects of the long term use of psychotropic drugs, in J. Gabe and P. Williams (eds) *Tranquillisers: Social, Psychological and Clinical Perspectives*. London: Tavistock.

Henderson, S. (1992) Living with the virus: Perspectives from HIV positive women in London, in N. Dorn and S. Hender (eds) *AIDS: Women, Drugs and Social Care*. London: Falmer Press.

Hepburn, M. (1992) Pregnancy and HIV: Screening, counselling and services, in J. Bury, V. Morrison and S. McLachlan (eds) *Working with Women and AIDS*. London: Routledge.

Herrero, R. *et al.* (1990) Injectable contraceptives and risk of invasive cervical cancer: evidence of an association. *International Journal of Cancer*, 46, 1, 5–7.

Hewitt, H. (1989) Correspondence. *British Medical Journal*, 299, 1337.

Hillan, E. M. (1992) Research and audit: Women's views of Caesarian sections, in H. Roberts (ed.) *Women's Health Matters*. London: Routledge.

Holland, J., Ramazanoglu, C., Scott, S., Sharpe, S. and Thomson, R. (1990a) *'Don't Die of Ignorance' – I nearly died of embarrassment. Condoms in Context. WRAP Paper 2*. London: The Tufnell Press.

Holland, J., Ramazanoglu, C. and Scott, S. (1990b) *Danger: AIDS Education Policy and Young Women's Sexuality. WRAP Paper 1*. London: The Tufnell Press.

Holland, J., Ramazanoglu, C., Sharpe, S. and Thomson, R. (1992) *Pressured Pleasure: Young Women and the Negotiation of Sexual Boundaries. WRAP Paper 7*. London: The Tufnell Press.

Horder, J. (1991) Long-term tranquilliser use: A general practitioner's view, in J. Gabe (ed.) *Understanding Tranquilliser Use*. London: Tavistock/Routledge.

Hornstein, F. (1984) Children by donor insemination: A new choice for lesbians, in R. Arditti, R. Klein and S. Minden (eds) *Test-Tube Women*. London: Pandora Press.

Horton, R. (1994) Trials of women. *The Lancet*, 343, 745–6.

House of Commons Health Committee (1991) *Second Report, Maternity Services,* vol. 1, House of Commons session 1991–92. London: HMSO.

Howarth, K. (1991) Are antenatal tests unhealthy? *GP,* 3 May, 56–7.

Hsu, L. K. (1986) The treatment of anorexia nervosa. *American Journal of Psychiatry,* 143, 573–81.

Hull, M. *et al.* (1992) Expectations of assisted conception for infertility. *British Medical Journal,* 304, 1465–9.

Hulley, S., Walsh, J. M. B. and Newman, T. B. (1992) Health policy on blood cholesterol: Time to change direction. *Circulation,* 86 (3), 1026–8.

Hunter, M., Battersby, R. and Whitehead, M. (1986) Relationship between psychological symptoms, somatic complaints and menopausal status. *Maturities,* 8, 217–28.

Hussey, H. H. (1974) Anorexia nervosa: Treatment by behaviour modification. *Journal of the American Medical Association,* 228, 344.

Hynes, P. and Spallone, P. (1990) 30 years of the pill. *Spare Rib,* 214, July, 48–9.

Illich, I. (1975) *Medical Nemesis: The Expropriation of Health.* London: Marion Boyars.

Illich, I. (1977) *Limits to Medicine.* Harmondsworth: Penguin.

Jacobs, H. S. and Loeffler, F. E. (1992) Postmenopausal hormone replacement therapy. *British Medical Journal,* 305, 1403–8.

Jacobson, B. (1981) *The Ladykillers.* 2nd edn. London: Pluto Press.

Jacobson, B. (1988) *Beating the Ladykillers.* London: Gollancz.

Jeffcoate, N. (1957) *Principles of Gynaecology.* London: Butterworth and Co.

Jennett, B. (1986) *High Technology Medicine: Benefits and Burdens.* Oxford: Oxford University Press.

Kahn, A. and Holt, L. H. (1989) *Menopause.* London: Bloomsbury.

Kane, P. (1991) *Women's Health: From Womb to Tomb.* London: Macmillan.

Kaplan, H. (1974) *The New Sex Therapy.* New York: Brunner Mazel.

Kimbrough, R. A. (1965) *Gynecology.* Philadelphia PA: Lippincott.

Kitzinger, S. (1979) *The Good Birth Guide.* London: Croom Helm.

Klein, R. (1984) Doing it ourselves: Self insemination, in R. Arditti, R. Klein and S. Minden (eds) *Test-Tube Women.* London: Pandora Press.

Klein, R. (1985) What's 'new' about the 'new' reproductive technologies?, in G. Corea *et al. Man Made Women.* London: Hutchinson.

Klein, R. (1989) *Infertility.* London: Pandora Press.

Klein, R. (1993) The NHS: Church or garage?, in A. Harrison (ed.) *Health Care UK, 1992/93.* London: King's Fund Institute.

Klemi, P. J., Joensuu, H., Toikkanen, S., Tuominen, J., Rasanen, O., Tyrkko, J. and Parvinen, I. (1992) Aggressiveness of breast cancers found with and without screening. *British Medical Journal,* 304, 467–9.

Knupfer, G. (1991) Abstaining for foetal health: The fiction that even light drinking is dangerous. *British Journal of Addiction,* 86, 1063–73.

Kolder, V., Gallaghar, J. and Parsons, M. (1987) Court ordered obstetrical interventions. *New England Journal of Medicine,* 316, 1192–6.

Lamb, B. (1987) Giving birth to the new-tech babies. *The Times,* 27 August.

Lasker, J. and Borg, S. (1989) *In Search of Parenthood.* London: Pandora Press.

The Lancet (1987) Editorial: Human papilloma viruses and cervical cancer: A fresh look at the evidence, 1 (8535), 725–6.

The Lancet (1989) Editorial: Is cervical laser therapy painful? 1(8628), 83.

The Lancet (1989) Editorial: Cerebral palsy, intrapartum care and a shot in the foot, II (8674), 1251–2.

Le Fanu, J. (1987) *Eat Your Heart Out*. London: Papermac.

Leeds Revolutionary Feminist Group (1982) Political lesbianism: The case against heterosexuality, in M. Evans (ed.) *The Woman Question*. London: Fontana.

Leiberman, J., Mazor, M., Chaim, W. and Cohen, A. (1979) The fetal right to live. *Obstetrics and Gynecology*, 53 (4), 515–17.

Leila, H. and Elliot, P. (1987) *Infertility and In Vitro Fertilisation*. London: BMA: Family Doctors Publication.

Levendusky, P. and Dooley, C. (1985) An inpatient model for the treatment of anorexia nervosa, in S. W. Emmett (ed.) *Theory and Treatment of Anorexia Nervosa and Bulimia*. New York: Brunner/Mazel.

Levin, A. (1991) The Angela Levin interview: Robert Winston, *The Mail on Sunday: You Magazine*, 8 December.

Lieberman, S. (1977) But you'll make such a feminine corpse. *Majority Report*, 19 February–4 March, 3–4.

Lilford, R. (1993) Infertility help 'more urgent than cancer therapy'. *The Guardian*, 11 May.

Lipsky, J. (1994) Concorde Lands. *The Lancet*, 343, 866–7.

Lister, S. (1984) Depo Provera – It can't end here. *WHIC Newsletter*, 3, 13–14.

Lopez-Jones, N. (ed.) (1992) *Prostitute Women and AIDS: Resisting the Virus of Repression*. London: Crossroads Books.

Loudon, N. (ed.) (1985) *Handbook of Family Planning*. Edinburgh: Churchill Livingstone.

Lovestone, S. and Fahy, T. (1991) Psychological factors in breast cancer. *British Medical Journal*, 302, 1219–20.

Lund, C. J. (1961) An epitaph for cervical cancer. *Journal of the American Medical Association*, 175, 122–3.

Lundgren, B. (1988) Breast screening in Britain and Sweden. *British Medical Journal*, 297, 1266.

McCarthy, K. H., Johnson, M. A. and Studd, J. W. W. (1992) Antenatal HIV testing. *British Journal of Obstetrics and Gynaecology*, 99, 867–8.

McConville, B. (1983) *Women Under the Influence: Alcohol and its Impact*. London: Virago.

McCormick, J. (1989) Cervical smears: A questionable practice? *The Lancet*, II (8656), 207–9.

McDonnell, K. (1988) Saying no to amnio. *Healthsharing*, Autumn, 23–4.

MacFarlane, A. and Mugford, A. (1986) An epidemic of Caesareans? (Part 2). *Maternity Alliance*, 25, July – August, 6.

MacIver, N. (1992) Developing a service for prostitutes in Glasgow, in J. Bury, V. Morrison and S. McLachlan (eds) *Working with Women and AIDS*. London: Routledge.

McKee, I. (1984) Community ante-natal care: The Sighthill Community Antenatal Scheme, in L. Zander and G. Chamberlain (eds) *Pregnancy Care for the 1980s*. London: The Royal Society of Medicine and Macmillan Press.

McKeganey, N., Barnard, M., Leyland, A., Coote, I. and Follett, E. (1992) Female streetworking prostitution and HIV infection in Glasgow. *British Medical Journal*, 305, 801–4.

Macnaughton, M. (1991) in *Health Committee Second Report Maternity Services*, 3. London: HMSO, 816.

McNay, M. B. and Whitfield, C. R. (1984) Prenatal diagnosis: Amniocentesis. *British Journal of Hosptial Medicine*, 31, 406–16.

McPherson, A. and Savage, W. (1987) Cervical cytology, in A. McPherson (ed.) *Women's Problems in General Practice*. 2nd edn. Oxford: Oxford University Press.

McTaggart, L. (1990) Screen violence. *What Doctors Don't Tell You*, 1 (6), 1–3.

McTaggart, L. (1991a) Dead certainty. *What Doctors Don't Tell You*, 2, (6), 1–3.

McTaggart, L. (1991b) The smear campaign. *What Doctors Don't Tell You*, 1, (3).

McTaggart, L. (1993) Breast cancer: The unkindest cut. *What Doctors Don't Tell You*, 3, (11), 1–3.

Maddocks, L. (1987) Minor tranx: No thanks. *Open Mind*, 29, 16–17.

Marx, S. (1990) Desire cannot be fragmented. *Connexions*, 33, 6–9.

Mason, V. (1989) *Women's Experiences of Maternity Care – A Survery Manual*. London: HMSO.

Masters, W. H. and Johnson, V. E. (1988) *Crisis: Heterosexual Behaviour in the Age of AIDS*. London: Weidenfeld and Nicholson.

Mauro, J. (1994) And Prozac for all. *Psychology Today*, 27(4), 44–8.

Melville, A. and Johnson, C. (1983) *Cured to Death*. Sevenoaks: New English Library.

Melville, J. (1984) *The Tranquilliser Trap and How to Get Out of It*. London: Fontana.

Menning, B. E. (1981) In defence of in-vitro fertilization, in H. B. Holmes, B. B. Hoskins and M. Gross (eds), *The Custom-Made Child? Women Centred Perspectives*. Clifton: Humana Press.

The Mental Health Foundation (1993) *Mental Illness: The Fundamental Facts*. London: Mental Health Foundation.

Miles, A. (1988) *Women and Mental Illness*. Brighton: Wheatsheaf Books.

Millar, J. (1992) Lone mothers and poverty, in C. Glendinning and J. Millar (eds) *Women and Poverty in Britain in the 1990s*. London: Harvester Wheatsheaf.

Modan, B. (1992) Diet and cancer: Causal relation or just wishful thinking? *The Lancet*, 340, 162–3.

Monk, J. (1990) 'Recovery from anorexia nervosa: A study of treatment'. Unpublished MSc thesis, University of Manchester.

Montsho, M. (1991) The dental dam fights back. *Spare Rib*, February, 58.

Moore, W. (1992) High hopes. *Health Service Journal*, 23 July, 10–11.

Moran, M. (1994) 'Three faces of the health care state'. Unpublished paper, Department of Government, University of Manchester.

Mosse, J. and Heaton, J. (1990) *The Fertility and Contraception Book*. London: Faber and Faber.

Mundy, B. (1988) Cervical cancer. *Spare Rib*, 187, 25–7.

National Childbrith Trust (NCT) (1975) *Some Mothers' Experiences of Induced Labour*. London: NCT.

National Childbirth Trust (NCT) (1989) *Rupture of the Membranes in Labour*. London: NCT.

National Childbirth Trust (NCT) (1991) *Memorandum to the House of Commons Health Committee*. HC (1990–91) 430–11.

National Institute of Health (1979) Report of the working group to review the NCI/ACS breast cancer detection project. *Journal of the National Cancer Institute*, 62, 641–709.

Neville-Lister, C. (1993) in L. R. Pembroke (ed.) *Eating Distress: Perspectives from Personal Experience*. Chartridge Chesham: Survivors Speak Out.

New Woman, April 1992, 38–44.

Newnham, J. P., Evans, S. F., Michael, C. A., Stanley, F. J. and Landau, L. I. (1993) Effects of frequent ultrasound during pregnancy: A randomised controlled trial. *The Lancet*, 342, 887–91.

Norton, R., Batey, R., Dwyer, T. and MacMahon, S. (1987) Alcohol consumption and the risk of related cirrhosis in women. *British Medical Journal*, 295, 80–2.

Novak, E. R. (1956) *Textbook of Gynaecology*. London: Balliere and Tindall.

Oakley, A. (1980) *Women Confined: Towards a Sociology of Childbirth*. Oxford: Martin Robertson.

Oakley, A. (1989) Smoking in pregnancy: Smokescreen or risk factor? Towards a materialist analysis. *Sociology of Health and Illness*, 11(4), 311–35.

Oakley, A. (1993) *Essays on Women, Medicine and Health*, Edinburgh: Edinburgh University Press.

Office of Health Economics (1987) *Women's Health Today*. London: Office of Health Economics.

Oliver, M. (1992) Doubts about preventing coronary heart disease. *British Medical Journal*, 304, 393–4.

Oxford Women's Health Action Group. (1984) *Whose Choice? What Women Have to Say About Contraception*. Oxford: Oxford Women's Health Action Group.

Padian, N. (1988) Prostitute women and AIDS: Epidemiology. *AIDS*, 2, 413–9.

Page, H. (1989) Calculating the effectiveness of in-vitro fertilisation: A review. *British Journal of Obstetrics and Gynaecology*, 96(3), 334–9.

Palmer, J. (1991) How sick can you get? *Daily Mirror*, 25 September, 2–3.

The Panos Institute (1990) *Triple Jeopardy: Women and AIDS*. London: Panos Publications.

Patton, C. (1990) *Inventing AIDS*. London: Routledge.

Paul, C., Skegg, D. C. G. and Spears, G. F. S. (1989) Depot Medroxyprogesterone (Depo-Provera) and risk of breast cancer. *British Medical Journal*, 299, 759–62.

Pembroke, L. R. (1993) *Eating Disorders: Perspectives from Personal Experience*. Chartridge Chesham: Survivors Speak Out.

Pequignot, G., Chabret, C., Eydoux, H. and Courcoul, M. A. (1974) Augmentation du risque de cirrhose en fonction de la ration d'alcool. *Revue de l'Alcolisme*, 20, 191–202.

Phillips, A. and Rakusen, J. (eds), (1989) *The New Our Bodies, Ourselves*. London: Penguin.

Pike, M. (1988) in L. Hodgkinson, Elixir of youth? *Women's Journal*, September 1988, 65–72.

Pike, M. C., Henderson, B. E., Krailo, M. D. and Duke, A. (1983) Breast cancer in young women and the use of oral contraceptives: possible modifying effect of formulation and age at use. *The Lancet*, 8356, 926–9.

Pippard, J. (1992) Audit of electroconvulsive treatment in two National Health Service regions. *British Journal of Psychiatry*, 160, 621–37.

Plant, M. (1987) *Women, Drinking and Pregnancy*. London: Tavistock.

Platt, S. (1991) Fertility Control. *New Statesman and Society*, 4(157), 11.

Pollitt, K. (1990) A new assault on feminism. *The Nation*, 26 March.

Pollock, S. (1984) Refusing to take women seriously: 'side effects' and the politics of contraception, in R. Arditti *et al.* (eds.) *Test-Tube Women*. London: Pandora Press.

Posner, T. and Vessey, M. (1988) *Prevention of Cervical Cancer: The Patients' View*. London: Edwards' Hospital Fund for London.

Prather, J. E. (1991) Decoding advertising: The role of communication studies in explaining the popularity of minor tranquillisers, in J. Gabe. (ed.) *Understanding Tranquilliser Use*. London: Tavistock/Routledge.

Prentice, A. and Lind, T. (1987) Fetal heart rate monitoring during labour – Too frequent intervention. Too little benefit? *The Lancet*, 8572, 1375–7.

Priest, R. G. (1989) Antidepressants of the future. *British Journal of Psychiatry*, 155 (suppl. 6), 7–8.

Quick, A. and Wilkinson, R. (1991) *Income and Health*. London: Socialist Health Association.

Quilligan, E. and Paul, R. (1975) Fetal monitoring: Is it worth it? *Obstetrics and Gynecology*, 45, January–June, 96–100.

Rakusen, J. (1990) *HIV and AIDS: What all Women Need to Know*. Manchester: North West Regional Health Authority.

Ramsay, L., Yeo, W., Jackson, P. (1991) Dietary reduction of serum cholesterol concentration: Time to think again. *British Medical Journal*, 303, 953–7.

Randhawa, K. (1986) Late booking – whose problem is it? *Maternity Action*, July–August, 9.

Rappoport, J. (1988) *AIDS Incorporated: Scandal of the Century*. San Bruno CA: Human Energy Press.

Ray, L. (1991) The political economy of long-term minor tranquilliser use, in J. Gabe (ed.) *Understanding Tranquilliser Use*. London: Tavistock/Routledge.

Raymond, J. (1984) Feminist ethics, ecology and vision, in R. Arditti, R. Klein and S. Minden (eds.), *Test-Tube Women*. London: Pandora Press.

Raymond, J. (1991) RU 486: A Medical Miracle? *Spare Rib*, 220, 34–7.

Redmayne, S. and Klein, R. (1993) Rationing practice: The case of in-vitro fertilisation. *British Medical Journal*, 306, 1521–4.

Reid, K. (1985) Choice of method, in N. Loudon (ed.) *Handbook of Family Planning*. Edinburgh: Churchill Livingstone.

Reitz, R. (1985) *Menopause: A Positive Approach*. London: Allen & Unwin.

Richards, T. (1989) Breast cancer screening in Britain. *British Medcial Journal*, 299, 877–8.

Richardson, D. (1989) *Women and the AIDS Crisis*. London: Pandora.

Roberts, H. (1985) *The Patient Patients: Women and their Doctors*. London: Pandora Press.

Roberts, M. (1989) Breast screening: Time for a rethink? *British Medical Journal*, 299, 1153–5.

Roberts, M. *et al.* (1990) Edinburgh trial of screening for breast cancer: mortality at seven years. *The Lancet*, 335, 241–6.

Robertson, J. (1989) Ethical and legal issues in human egg donation. *Fertility and Sterility*, 52(3), 353–62.

Robinson, J. (1981) Cervical cancer: A feminist critique. *Times Health Supplement*. 27 November.

Robinson, J. (1984) Promiscuity isn't the cause. *New Statesman*, 30 March.

Robinson, J. (1988) *Jancis Robinson on the Demon Drink*. London: Mitchell Beazley.

Rodgers, A. (1991) Letter in *British Medical Journal*, 302, 1401.

Rogers, L. (1993) Row over human eggs 'for sale'. *The Sunday Times*, 28 March.

Roland, N. (1990) *Sex Rules*. Manchester: North West Regional Health Authority.

Romanis, R. (1987) *Depression*. London: Faber and Faber.

Rosenwaks, Z. (1987) Donor eggs: Their application in modern reproductive technologies. *Fertility and Sterility*. 47(6), 895–909.

Ross, S. K. (1989) Cervical cytology screening and government policy. *British Medical Journal*, 299, 101–4.

Rothman, B. (1984) The meanings of choice in reproductive technology, in R. Arditti, R. Klein and S. Minder (eds.) *Test-Tube Women*. London: Pandora Press.

Rowe, D. (1991) *Breaking the Bonds*. London: Fontana.

Rowland, R. (1992) *Living Laboratories*. London: Cedar.

Royal College of General Practitioners/Royal College of Gynaecologists (RCGP/RCOG) (1985) Induced abortion operations and their early sequelae. *Journal of the Royal College of General Practitioners*, 35, 175–80.

Royal College of Obstetricians and Gynaecologists (RCOG) (1983) *Report of the RCOG Ethics Committee on In Vitro Fertilisation and Embryo Replacement or Transfer*. London: RCOG.

Royal College of Obstetricians and Gynaecologists (RCOG) (1991) in House of Commons Health Committee *Second Report, Maternity Services*, xivii. London: HMSO.

Royal College of Physicians (1987) *A Great and Growing Evil: The Medical Consequences of Alcohol Abuse*. London: Tavistock.

Royal College of Psychiatrists. (1986) *Alcohol: Our Favourite Drug*. London: Tavistock.

Rutter, D. Calnan, M., Vaile, M., Field, S. and Wade, K. (1992) Discomfort and pain during mammography: Description prediction and prevention. *British Medical Journal*, 305, 443–5.

Sack, F. (1992) *Romance to Die For*. Deerfield Beach, FL: Health Communications Inc.

Saffron, L. (1984) Caps – old and new. *WHIC Newsletter*, 2, Spring.

Salvesen, K. A., Vatten, L. J., Eik-Nes, S. H., Hugdahl, K. and Bakketeig, L. S. (1993) Routine ultrasonography in utero and subsequent handedness and neurological development. *British Medical Journal*, 307, 159–64.

Savage, W., Schwartz, M. and George, J. (1989) 'A survey of women's knowledge, attitudes and experience of cervical screening in the Tower Hamlets Health District'. Unpublished report.

Schoener, G., Hofstee, M. and Gonsiorek, J. (1984) Sexual exploitation of clients by therapists. *Women and Mental Health*, 3, 63–9.

Scutt, J. (ed.), (1988) *The Baby Machine*. Melbourne: McCulloch Publishing.

Seaman, B. (1978) The Dangers of Sex Hormones, in C. Dreifus (ed.) *Seizing Our Bodies*. New York: Vintage Books.

Secretary of State for Health. (1991) *The Health of the Nation*, Cm. 1523. London: HMSO.

Shapiro, J. (1987) Menopause – Growing old in a man's world, in S. O'Sullivan (ed.) *Women's Health: A Spare Rib Reader*. London: Pandora.

Shapiro, R. (1987) *Contraception: A Practical and Political Guide*. London: Virago.

Shaw, W. (1956) *Textbook of Gynaecology*. 7th edn. London: J and A Churchill.

Shearer, B. (1989) Forced Caesareans: the case of the disappearing mother. *International Journal of Childbirth Education*, 4(1), 7–10.

Shorter, E. (1984) *A History of Women's Bodies*. Harmondsworth: Penguin Books.

Showalter, E. (1987) *The Female Malady*. London: Virago.

Skrabanek, P. (1987) Cervical cancer screening. *The Lancet*, 1(8547) 1432.

Skrabanek, P. (1988a). Cervical cancer in nuns and prostitutes: A plea for scientific continence. *Journal of Clinical Epidemiology*, 41(6), 577–82.

Skrabanek, P. (1988b) The debate over mass mammography in Britain: The case against. *British Medical Journal*, 297, 971–2.

Skrabanek, P. (1990) Breast cancer screening. *Update*, 15 March, 627–9.

Skrabanek, P. and McCormick, J. (1989) *Follies and Fallacies in Medicine*. Glasgow: The Tarragon Press.

Smith, A., Elkind, A. and Eardley, A. (1989) Making cervical screening work, *British Medical Journal*, 298, 1662–4.

Smith, R. (ed.) (1991) *The Health of the Nation: The BMJ View*. London: British Medical Journal.

Spallone, P. (1989) *Beyond Conception*. Basingstoke: Macmillan.

Spring-Rice, M. (1981) *Working Class Wives*. 2nd edn. London: Virago.

Springer, E. (1992) Reflections on women and HIV/AIDS in New York City and the United States, in J. Bury, V. Morrison and S. McLachlan (eds) *Working with Women and AIDS*. London: Tavistock/ Routledge.

Stanworth, M. (1987) Reproductive technologies and the deconstruction of motherhood, in M. Stanworth (ed.) *Reproductive Technologies*. Cambridge: Polity Press.

Statham, H. (1987) Cold comfort. *The Guardian*, 1 March.

Statham, J. and Green, J. (1993) Serum screening for Down's Syndrome: Some women's experiences. *British Medical Journal*, 307, 174–6.

Steer, P. (1993) Rituals in ante-natal care – do we need them? *British Medical Journal*, 307, 697–8.

Steinberg, K., Thacker, S. B., Jay Smith, S., Stroup, D. F., Zack, M. M., Flanders, D. and Berkelman, R. L. (1991) A meta-analysis of the effect of estrogen replacement therapy on the risk of breast cancer. *Journal of the American Medical Association*, 265(15), 1985–90.

Stellman, J. and Bertin, J. (1990) Science's Anti-female Bias. *The New York Times*, 4 June.

Stewart, G. (1992) AIDS, the myths and the martyrdom. *The Daily Mail*, 5 April.

Stewart, H. (1988) Are two views better than one? The research continues. *New Scientist*, 15 October, 51.

Storey, P. (1986) *Psychological Medicine: An Introduction to Psychiatry*. 10th edn. Edinburgh: Churchill Livingstone.

Stott, P. (1991) Implications for practice budgets of increasing numbers of HRT prescriptions. *Well Woman Team*, 1(4), 2–3.

Studd, J. (1988) in L. Hodgkinson Elixir of Youth? *Women's Journal*, September, 65–72.

Tabar, L. *et al.* (1988) The results of periodic one-view mammography screening in a randomised control trial in Sweden, in N. Day and A. Miller (eds) *Screening for Breast Cancer*. Toronto: Huber.

Taylor, A. (1992) It felt as though he had seduced me. *The Independent*, 1 September.

Taylor, P. J. (1990) When is enough enough? *Fertility and Sterility*, 54(5), 772–4.

Taylor, R. (1979) *Medicine Out of Control*. Melbourne: Sun Books.

Tew, M. (1991) Supplementary memorandum submitted by Mrs Marjorie Tew, in *House of Commons Health Committee Second Report*, Vol. II, Minutes of Evidence. London: HMSO, 580–91.

Thomas, D. B. and Ray, R. M. (1992) Depot-Medroxyprogesterone Acetate (DMPA) and risk of invasive squamus cell cervical cancer. *Contraception*, 45(4), 299–312.

Thomas, R. M. (1992) HIV and the sex industry, in J. Bury, V. Morrison and S. McLachlan (eds) *Working with Women and AIDS*. London: Routledge.

Thomson, K. (1992) Being positive, in J. Bury, V. Morrison and S. McLachlan (eds.) *Working with Women and AIDS*. London: Routledge.

Tindall, V. R. (1987) *Jeffcoate's Principles of Gynaecology*. 5th edn. London: Butterworth.

Treffers, P. and Pel, M. (1993) The rising trend for caesarian birth. *British Medical Journal*, 307, 1017–8.

Tulandi, T. and Cherry, N. (1989) Clinical trials in reproductive surgery: randomization and life-table analysis. *Fertility and Sterility*, 52(1), 12–14.

Tyrer, P. (1988) Benefits and risks of benzodiazepines, in H. Freeman and Y. Rue (eds) *The Benzodiazepines in Current Clinical Practice*. London: Royal Society of Medicine Services.

Tyrer, P. and Murphy, S. (1987) The place of benzodiazepines in psychiatric practice. *British Journal of Psychiatry*, 151, 719–23.

Ussher, J. (1989) *The Psychology of the Female Body*. London: Routledge.

Ussher, J. (1991) *Women's Madness: Misogyny or Mental Illness?*. London: Harvester Wheatsheaf.

Vandenbroucke, J. P. (1991) Postmenopausal oestrogen and cardio-protection. *The Lancet*, 337, 833–4.

Wagner, M. and St Clair, P. A. (1989) Are in-vitro fertilisation and embryo transfer of benefit to all? *The Lancet*, II, (8670), 1027–8.

Walker, A. (1992) The poor relation: Poverty among older women, in C. Glendinning and J. Millar (eds) *Women and Poverty in Britain in the 1990s*. London: Harvester Wheatsheaf.

Warnock, M. (1985) *A Question of Life*. Oxford: Basil Blackwell.

Warren, R. (1988) The debate over mass mammography in Britain: The case for. *British Medical Journal*, 297, 969–70.

Weideger, P. (1976) *Female Cycles: Menstruation and Menopause*. London: Women's Press.

Wells, J. and Batten, L. (1990) Women's smoking and coping: An analysis of women's experiences of stress. *Health Education Journal*, 49(2), 57–60.

Wharton, L. (1943) *Gynecology*. Philadelphia: W. B. Saunders.

Wheble, A., Gillmer, M. D. G., Spencer, J. A. D. and Sykes, G. S (1989) Changes in fetal monitoring practice in the UK: 1977–1984. *British Journal of Obstetrics and Gynaecology*, 96, 1140–7.

White, P. (1987) Women and smoking, in A. McPherson (ed.) *Women's Problems in General Practice*. Oxford: Oxford University Press.

Willet, W. (1989) The search for the causes of breast and colon cancer. *Nature*, 338, 389–93.

Wilson, E. S. (1985) Injectable contraceptives, in N. Loudon (ed.) *Handbook of Family Planning*. Edinburgh: Churchill Livingstone.

Wilson, J. (1992) Offering safer sex counselling to women from drug-using communities, in J. Bury, V. Morrison and S. McLachlan (eds) *Working with Women and AIDS*. London: Tavistock/Routledge.

Wilson, R. (1966) *Feminine Forever*. London: W.H. Allen.

Wilton, T. (1992) *Anti-body Politic: AIDS and Society*. Cheltenham: New Clarion Press.

Winn, M. (1991) The grim reaper: Australia's first mass media AIDS education campaign, in World Health Organisation, *AIDS Prevention Through Health Promotion*. Geneva: WHO.

Winston, R. (1985) Why we need to experiment. *The Observer*, 10 February.

Winston, R. and Margara, R. (1987) Letter in *British Medical Journal*, 295, 785.

Witcombe, J. (1988) A licence for breast cancer screening? *British Medical Journal*, 296, 909–12.

Worcester, N. and Whatley, M. (1992) The selling of HRT: Playing on the fear factor. *Feminist Review*, 41, 1–26.

Wright, J. T. (1989) Is cervical laser therapy painful? *The Lancet*, 8688, 335.

Yanoshik, K. and Norsigian, J. (1989) Contraception, control and choice: International perspectives, in K. S. Ratcliff (ed.) *Healing Technology: Feminist Perspectives.* Ann Arbor: The University of Michigan Press.

Younger, J. (1989). Truth in advertising. *Fertility and Sterility.* 52(5), 726–7.

Yudkin, G. (1984) A month in the life of a general practitioner – or how the pill scare wasn't scary enough. *WHIC Newsletter*, 2, Spring.

INDEX

GRIMSBY COLLEGE LIBRARY NUNS CORNER, GRIMSBY